MEDITERRANEAN DIET COOKBOOK FOR BEGINNERS: HEALTHY AND SUPER-EASY EVERYDAY MEDITERRANEAN RECIPES.

By
Sophia Bexley

TABLE OF CONTENTS

INTRODUCTION

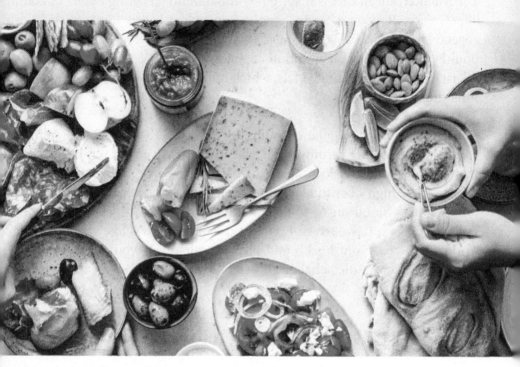

⁷hat if you could bring the vibrant, sun-soaked flavors of the Mediterranean
ht into your kitchen while boosting your health along the way? The
:diterranean diet is a lifestyle that focuses on wholesome ingredients like
:sh vegetables, lean proteins, and whole grains, balanced with heart-healthy
s. It's celebrated for its ability to boost energy, improve well-being, and deliver
icious meals you'll look forward to every day.

is cookbook brings you an exciting variety of Mediterranean-inspired
hes. From refreshing breakfast options to flavorful appetizers and snacks,
:h dish is designed to be both simple and satisfying. Explore colorful
;etable recipes and comforting soups that bring warmth to the table.
lulge in hearty pasta and pizza for a true Mediterranean experience, or
out protein-rich poultry and meat dishes that are sure to impress. If you
e seafood, you'll appreciate the fresh fish and seafood recipes that capture
essence of coastal cuisine. And, of course, end your meal with sweet and
isfying desserts. Whether you're an experienced cook or a beginner, these
ipes will effortlessly bring the Mediterranean way of eating to your kitchen.

What is the Mediterranean Diet

The Mediterranean diet is inspired by the traditional eating habits of countri
like Greece, Italy, and Spain, emphasizing plant-based foods such as frui
vegetables, whole grains, legumes, and nuts, with moderate intake of fish a
poultry and limited consumption of red meat. A key feature is the use of oli
oil, rich in monounsaturated fats, which improves cholesterol levels and reduc
inflammation.

The diet encourages regular consumption of omega-3-rich fish like salmon a
sardines, supporting cardiovascular health. Extensive research has shown th
this diet lowers the risk of heart disease, stroke, type 2 diabetes, and certa
cancers. The high fiber intake from whole grains and vegetables aids digesti
and regulates blood sugar, while antioxidants in fruits, vegetables, and olive
help combat oxidative stress. Fermented dairy products like yogurt and chee
also contribute to gut health and provide calcium for bone strength, maki
the Mediterranean diet a balanced, scientifically-backed approach to long-te
health.

History of the Mediterranean Diet

The history of the Mediterranean diet dates back thousands of years, rooted
the agricultural practices, social traditions, and culinary habits of civilizatic
surrounding the Mediterranean Sea. Ancient Greek, Roman, and Egypti
communities developed diets based on locally available ingredients such
grains, olives, and grapes. These crops thrived in the Mediterranean clima
characterized by mild, wet winters and hot, dry summers, which allowed for
cultivation of wheat, barley, olive trees, and vineyards. Olive oil, in particu
became a staple in both culinary and cultural practices, serving not only a
key food item but also for medicinal, religious, and trade purposes. Along w
olives, grains like wheat and barley were ground into bread, forming the base
daily sustenance, often accompanied by wine, fish, and vegetables, while m
was consumed less frequently due to its scarcity and cost.

The concept of the Mediterranean diet as a formalized nutritional patt
gained recognition in the mid-20th century, following the work of Ameri
scientist Ancel Keys. In the 1950s, Keys conducted the Seven Countries Stu
which examined the dietary habits and health outcomes of populations

eece, Italy, and other nations. He observed that people in Mediterranean
gions, particularly on the Greek island of Crete, exhibited significantly lower
es of heart disease and lived longer lives compared to those in countries
th diets higher in saturated fats, such as the U.S. and northern Europe. This
search highlighted the health benefits of the Mediterranean way of eating,
ich emphasized plant-based foods, healthy fats from olive oil, and moderate
nsumption of fish and poultry. Over time, Keys' findings and subsequent
dies led to the global promotion of the Mediterranean diet as a model for
althy living, recognized today by nutritionists and health organizations as one
the most beneficial diets for long-term health.

Mediterranean Diet

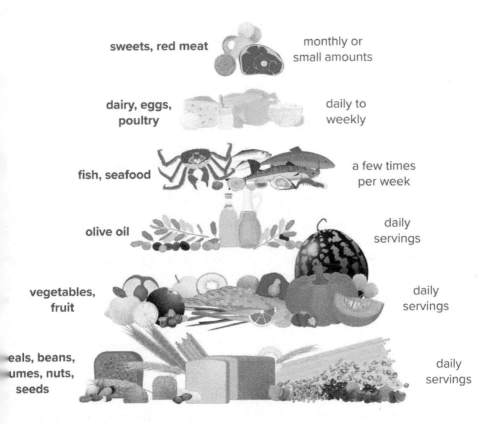

: Mediterranean diet is one of the most researched and widely recommended
ary patterns for promoting long-term health and reducing the risk of chronic
ases. Rooted in the traditional eating habits of Mediterranean countries, it
hasizes whole, natural foods and a balanced approach to nutrition.

High Intake of Plant-Based Foods

The Mediterranean diet prioritizes plant-based foods such as fruits, vegetabl legumes, whole grains, nuts, and seeds.

- Rich in fiber, promoting healthy digestion and improving gut health.
- High in vitamins and minerals, supporting immune function and over vitality.
- Antioxidants from fruits and vegetables reduce oxidative stress a inflammation.
- Legumes and whole grains offer slow-digesting carbohydrates, stabiliz blood sugar levels.
- Nuts and seeds provide healthy fats and plant-based proteins, support heart health.

Olive Oil as the Primary Source of Fat

Olive oil, especially extra virgin olive oil, is a central component of Mediterranean diet. It is rich in monounsaturated fats and polyphenols, wh have numerous health benefits.

- Contains oleic acid, which lowers LDL (bad) cholesterol and increa HDL (good) cholesterol.
- Rich in antioxidants like polyphenols, which protect cells from damag
- Anti-inflammatory properties help reduce the risk of chronic diseases heart disease.
- Promotes better blood sugar control, which can reduce the risk of typ diabetes.
- Supports brain health, with studies linking olive oil consumption improved cognitive function.

Regular Consumption of Fish and Seafood

Fish and seafood, particularly fatty fish like salmon, sardines, mackerel, anchovies, are rich in omega-3 fatty acids, which are essential for heart brain health.

- Omega-3s help lower triglycerides and prevent plaque buildup in arteries.
- Promotes better brain health, reducing the risk of cognitive decline dementia.

- Fatty fish provide high-quality protein with low saturated fat content.
- Fish contains essential nutrients like vitamin D and selenium, supporting overall health.
- Regular consumption reduces inflammation and the risk of chronic conditions, such as arthritis.

Moderate Dairy Consumption

The Mediterranean diet includes moderate amounts of dairy, primarily in the form of fermented products like yogurt and cheese, which are rich in probiotics and calcium.

- Fermented dairy promotes gut health by providing beneficial bacteria (probiotics).
- Calcium from yogurt and cheese supports bone density and prevents osteoporosis.
- Lower in lactose, fermented dairy is easier to digest for many people.
- Fermented dairy may improve cholesterol levels, unlike high-fat, unfermented dairy.
- It provides a source of protein and fat without excessive calories and fits into a balanced diet.

Fresh, Seasonal, and Local Ingredients

The Mediterranean diet places a strong emphasis on the use of fresh, seasonal, and locally sourced ingredients, which are not only more flavorful but also more nutrient-dense.

- Seasonal produce is harvested at peak ripeness, ensuring maximum nutrient content.
- Fresh ingredients are free from preservatives and additives commonly found in processed foods.
- Locally sourced foods reduce environmental impact by cutting down on transportation emissions.
- Eating seasonal foods supports local farmers and the regional economy.
- Fresh foods are less likely to be calorie-dense, contributing to better weight management.

Social and Mindful Eating Practices

A key element of the Mediterranean diet is the cultural practice of enjoying mea with family and friends, encouraging mindful eating and social connection.

- Sharing meals promotes emotional well-being and reduces stress.
- Mindful eating encourages slower, more deliberate consumptio improving digestion.
- Social interactions during meals are linked to lower rates of depressic and anxiety.
- Eating meals slowly helps prevent overeating and supports better weig control.
- The ritual of eating together fosters a stronger connection to food, creatii a healthier relationship with eating.

Foods Allowed

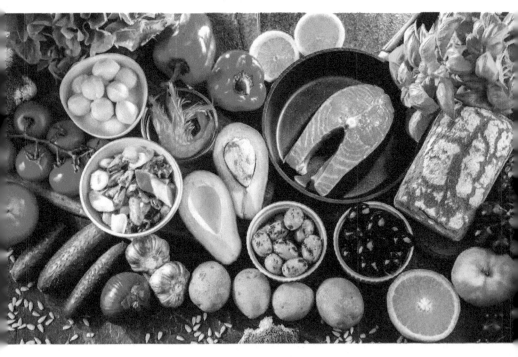

The Mediterranean diet is recognized for its balance, variety, and emphasis o nutrient-dense, whole foods. One of the key features of this diet is its flexibil: allowing for a wide range of foods in moderation rather than eliminating entire food groups.

Vegetables

Vegetables are at the core of the Mediterranean diet, and a wide variety is encouraged.

- Leafy Greens: Spinach, kale, Swiss chard, arugula, and lettuce.
- Cruciferous Vegetables: Broccoli, cauliflower, Brussels sprouts, and cabbage.
- Root Vegetables: Carrots, beets, turnips, sweet potatoes, and radishes.
- Nightshades: Tomatoes, eggplants, peppers, and zucchini.
- Alliums: Garlic, onions, leeks, and shallots.
- Squash and Gourds: Zucchini, pumpkin, and butternut squash.
- Fresh Herbs: Basil, parsley, cilantro, rosemary, thyme, and oregano (used to enhance flavor without adding unhealthy fats).

Fruits

Fresh, seasonal fruits are a major part of the Mediterranean diet, eaten as snacks desserts.

- Citrus Fruits: Oranges, lemons, grapefruits, and limes.
- Berries: Strawberries, blueberries, raspberries, blackberries, and grapes.
- Stone Fruits: Peaches, apricots, plums, cherries, and nectarines.
- Melons: Watermelon, cantaloupe, and honeydew.
- Pome Fruits: Apples and pears.
- Tropical Fruits: Figs, dates, and pomegranates (traditional in many Mediterranean dishes).
- Dried Fruits: Raisins, apricots, and figs (used in moderation, as they are calorie-dense).

Whole Grains and Cereals

Whole grains provide complex carbohydrates that fuel the body with long-lasting energy.

- Whole Wheat: Whole wheat bread, pasta, and bulgur.
- Rice: Brown rice and wild rice.
- Barley: Used in soups, stews, and salads.
- Quinoa: A complete protein and gluten-free grain alternative.
- Oats: Steel-cut or rolled oats for breakfast dishes and baking.

- Farro and Spelt: Ancient grains that are popular in Mediterranean dishes

Legumes and Beans

Rich in protein and fiber, legumes and beans are key to the plant-based nature of the diet.

- Chickpeas: Used in hummus, soups, and stews.
- Lentils: Brown, green, and red lentils in soups, stews, and salads.
- Beans: Kidney beans, black beans, cannellini beans, and fava beans.
- Peas: Split peas, green peas, and snow peas.

Fish and Seafood

Fatty fish is favored for its omega-3 content, but lean fish and shellfish are also widely consumed.

- Fatty Fish: Salmon, sardines, mackerel, anchovies, and trout.
- Lean Fish: Cod, sole, halibut, and sea bass.
- Shellfish: Shrimp, mussels, clams, oysters, and scallops.
- Squid and Octopus: Common in Mediterranean coastal regions, often grilled or stewed.

Poultry and Eggs

Poultry is consumed more often than red meat, and eggs are included regularly

- Chicken: Grilled, roasted, or stewed, often in Mediterranean spices and herbs.
- Turkey: Used in place of red meat in many dishes.
- Duck: Consumed occasionally.
- Eggs: Used in breakfast dishes, frittatas, and salads.

Dairy Products

Dairy is consumed in moderation, mostly from fermented sources.

- Yogurt: Plain Greek yogurt, rich in probiotics and protein.
- Cheese: Feta, goat cheese, ricotta, Parmesan, pecorino, and mozzarella
- Milk: Typically used in small quantities, with a preference for whole milk
- Kefir: A fermented dairy drink rich in probiotics.

d Meat

d meat is included to ensure a balanced intake of fats and proteins.

- Beef: Grass-fed beef is preferred for its lower fat content and healthier fat profile.
- Lamb: Common in Mediterranean dishes, often roasted or grilled.
- Pork: Used occasionally, often in small portions or as part of stews or roasts.

althy Fats

althy fats are crucial in the Mediterranean diet, particularly from plant-based rces.

- Olive Oil: Extra virgin olive oil for cooking, salad dressings, and drizzling.
- Avocados: Rich in monounsaturated fats and often added to salads and spreads.
- Nuts: Almonds, walnuts, pine nuts, pistachios, and hazelnuts (unsalted).
- Seeds: Flaxseeds, chia seeds, sesame seeds, and sunflower seeds.

rbs and Spices

sh and dried herbs and spices add flavor without the need for excess salt or healthy fats.

- Fresh Herbs: Basil, rosemary, thyme, oregano, parsley, and mint.
- Spices: Cumin, coriander, paprika, turmeric, cinnamon, and black pepper.
- Garlic and Onions: Essential for adding depth and flavor to many Mediterranean dishes.

ne (in moderation)

glass of red wine is often enjoyed with meals. Rich in antioxidants like reratrol, red wine is linked to heart health when consumed in moderation bically no more than one glass per day).

Nuts and Seeds

Nuts and seeds are a crucial source of healthy fats, protein, fiber, and essent
nutrients such as magnesium, zinc, and selenium. They are typically eaten r
or lightly toasted without added salt or sugar.

- Almonds: Rich in vitamin E and magnesium, commonly eaten as sna
  or used in cooking.
- Walnuts: High in omega-3 fatty acids, often used in salads or baking.
- Pine Nuts: A traditional ingredient in Mediterranean pesto and vari
  dishes.
- Pistachios: Often eaten as snacks or added to savory and sweet dishes.
- Sesame Seeds: Used in tahini (sesame paste) and sprinkled on salads
  baked goods.
- Flaxseeds: A rich source of fiber and omega-3s, commonly added
  yogurt, smoothies, or baked goods.
- Sunflower Seeds: High in vitamin E and selenium, used as toppings o
  granola.
- Chia Seeds: A good source of omega-3s, fiber, and protein, often addec
  smoothies or used to make chia pudding.

Herbs and Seasonings

Herbs and seasonings in the Mediterranean diet not only add flavor but a
provide health benefits, with many possessing antioxidant and anti-inflammat
properties.

- Basil: Fresh basil is often used in salads, sauces (like pesto), and as a garn
- Oregano: A key herb in Mediterranean cooking, used in marinades, ste
  and salads.
- Rosemary: Used to flavor meats, vegetables, and bread and has antioxid
  properties.
- Thyme: Common in Mediterranean soups, stews, and meat dishes.
- Mint: Fresh mint is often used in salads and teas and as a garnish
  various dishes.
- Coriander/Cilantro: Adds a fresh, zesty flavor to salads and cooked dis
- Parsley: Widely used for garnish and flavoring, as well as in tabbouleh
  sauces.
- Bay Leaves: Often added to soups, stews, and slow-cooked dishes for fla
- Sumac: A tangy, lemony spice often used in Middle Eastern Mediterran
  dishes.
- Paprika: Adds a smoky or spicy kick to meats, stews, and vegetables.
- Cumin: Common in Mediterranean and Middle Eastern dishes, especi
  in spice blends like za'atar.

Fermented Foods

Fermented foods provide probiotics, which help balance the gut microbiome, supporting digestive health and overall well-being.

- Kefir: A fermented milk drink that is rich in probiotics and calcium.
- Fermented Vegetables: Traditional Mediterranean cultures also enjoy pickled vegetables such as cucumbers, peppers, and cabbage.
- Olives: Not only used for oil but also consumed whole as fermented snacks, providing healthy fats and antioxidants.
- Sauerkraut: Though more commonly associated with Eastern Europe, sauerkraut is sometimes included in Mediterranean dishes, particularly in the Balkans.
- Fermented Fish: Some Mediterranean regions (especially coastal areas) consume fermented fish in small quantities for its probiotic and omega-3 content.

Seaweed and Marine Plants

While not as central as in some Asian diets, certain Mediterranean coastal cultures, especially in regions like Greece, consume seaweed for its iodine and mineral content.

- Nori: Often added to Mediterranean seafood dishes or salads.
- Kelp: Consumed in soups or as a garnish in coastal areas.

Beverages (Other than Wine)

While wine is the most iconic beverage in the Mediterranean diet, other beverages play a role in daily hydration and health.

- Water: Freshwater is the primary drink in the Mediterranean diet, often infused with herbs like mint or fruits like lemon for added flavor.
- Herbal Teas: Teas made from herbs such as chamomile, peppermint, and fennel are commonly consumed for digestive health and relaxation.
- Coffee: In moderate amounts, coffee is enjoyed across Mediterranean countries, typically black or with a small amount of milk, but without excessive sugar or cream.

Spreads and Pastes

Spreads and pastes are an integral part of Mediterranean meals, often used appetizers or accompaniments to other dishes.

- Hummus: A traditional spread made from blended chickpeas, tahini, oli oil, garlic, and lemon juice. It's rich in protein, fiber, and healthy fats.
- Baba Ganoush: A smoky eggplant-based spread, often served with p; bread or fresh vegetables.
- Tahini: A sesame seed paste that's a staple in Middle Eastern Mediterrane dishes, used in hummus, dressings, and desserts.
- Tapenade: A spread made from blended olives, capers, and anchovi typically served with bread or vegetables.
- Skordalia: A Greek garlic-based dip, often made with potatoes or bre; olive oil, and vinegar.

Bread

Bread in the Mediterranean diet is typically whole grain or made from ancie grains, eaten in moderation, and often dipped in olive oil rather than butter.

- Whole Wheat Bread: Made from 100% whole wheat, rich in fiber a nutrients.
- Pita Bread: A traditional flatbread, often used to scoop up dips l; hummus and baba ganoush.
- Sourdough Bread: A fermented bread that is easier to digest and lower the glycemic index than white bread.
- Focaccia: An Italian bread, often topped with herbs like rosemary a olive oil.
- Rye Bread: Popular in Mediterranean countries, especially in coastal a mountain regions.

Desserts

Desserts in the Mediterranean diet are enjoyed, often made from simple, natural ingredients like fruits, nuts, and honey.

- Fresh Fruit: Served as a dessert, either raw or lightly grilled with a drizzle of honey or balsamic vinegar.
- Baklava: A pastry made from layers of filo dough, honey, and nuts like pistachios or walnuts.
- Greek Yogurt with Honey and Nuts: A common, light dessert combining protein-rich yogurt with the natural sweetness of honey and the crunch of nuts.
- Fruit Compotes: Lightly stewed fruits, such as figs or apricots, often served with a dollop of yogurt.
- Torrone: A traditional Mediterranean nougat made with honey, sugar, egg whites, and nuts, such as almonds or pistachios.

Miscellaneous Foods

In addition to the core categories, several other foods are included in Mediterranean diets.

- Caper Berries: Often used in salads or to garnish seafood dishes, providing a briny, tangy flavor.
- Vinegar: Balsamic and red wine vinegars are used in salads and marinades, providing acidity without the need for excessive salt.
- Honey: Used sparingly as a natural sweetener in desserts and teas.
- Feta-Brined Vegetables: Certain vegetables like cucumbers and peppers may be brined or pickled with feta, a process popular in parts of Greece.

NOTES

BREAKFAST RECIPES

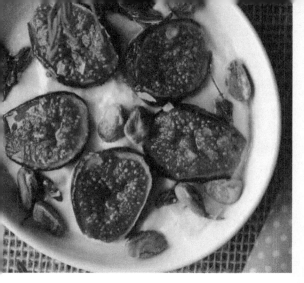

Yogurt & Fig Bowl

Prep period: 10 mins.
Cook period: 7 mins.
Serves: 4

Per Serving: Calories 296, Fat 3.8g
Carbs 58.8g, Protein 9.7g

INGREDIENTS REQUIRED:

- Honey – 3 tbsp. divided
- Fresh figs – 8 oz. (220 g), halved
- Plain Greek yogurt – 2 C. (500 g)
- Pistachios – ¼ C. (30 g), cut up

PROCEDURE:

1. Put 1 tbsp. of honey into a medium-sized wok on a burner at around medium heat.
2. Cook for around 1-2 minutes.
3. Put the figs into the wok cut side down.
4. Cook for around 5 minutes.
5. Take off the wok of figs from the burner and set it aside for around 2-3 minutes.
6. Divide the yogurt into serving dishes and top each with the caramelized fig halves.
7. Sprinkle with pistachios.
8. Drizzle each bowl with the remnant honeyand enjoy.

Dried Fruit Quinoa Porridge

Prep period: 10 mins.
Cook period: 20 mins.
Serves: 4

Per Serving: Calories 395, Fat 10.5g, Carbs 66.5g, Protein 9.9g

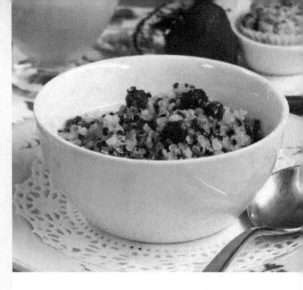

PROCEDURE:

- Put the quinoa and water into a large-sized pot on a burner at around medium heat.
- Cook the mixture until boiling.
- Turn the heat to around low.
- Cook with the cover for around 15 minutes, stirring from time to time.
- In the meantime, put the apricots, figs, walnuts, and cinnamon into a large-sized basin and blend thoroughly.
- Take off the pot of quinoa from the burner and, with a fork, fluff it.
- Put the quinoa into the basin of dried fruit mixture and toss to incorporate thoroughly.
- Divide the quinoa mixture into 4 mason jars and top each with milk.
- Cover the jars and put them into your fridge overnight before enjoying.

INGREDIENTS REQUIRED:

- Quinoa – 1 C. (190 g), rinsed
- Water – 2 C. (480 ml)
- Dried apricots – 8, cut into bite-sized pieces
- Dried figs – 8, cut into bite-sized pieces
- Walnuts – ¼ C. (25 g), cut up
- Ground cinnamon – 1 tsp.
- Whole milk – 2 C. (480 ml)

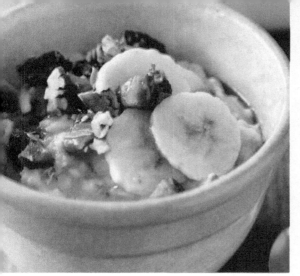

Barley Porridge

Prep period: 10 mins.
Cook period: 35 mins.
Serves: 4

Per Serving: Calories 452, Fat 9.1g,
Carbs 84.5g, Protein 13.7g

INGREDIENTS REQUIRED:

- Pearl barley – 1 C. (200 g)
- Whole milk – 3 C. (720 ml)
- Dried dates – ¼ C. (40 g), pitted and cut up
- Honey – ¼ C. (75 g)
- Small-sized bananas – 2, peel removed and sliced
- Walnuts – ¼ C. (25 g), cut up

PROCEDURE:

1. Put the water, barley, and dates into a large-sized pot on a burn at around medium-high heat.
2. Cook the mixture until boiling.
3. Turn the heat to around low.
4. Cook with the cover for around 25-30 minutes, stirring from tin to time.
5. Take off from the burner and blend in honey
6. Enjoy right away with the topping of banana slices and walnuts.

Tuna Omelet

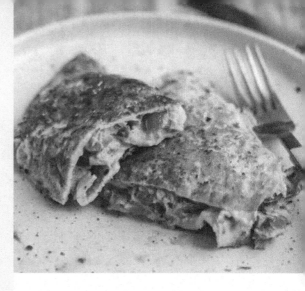

Prep period: 10 mins.

Cook period: 10 mins.

Serves: 4

Per Serving: Calories 172, Fat 11.6g, Carbs 3.1g, Protein 14.5g

PROCEDURE:

- Put the eggs, milk, Italian seasoning, salt, and pepper into a basin and whisk thoroughly. Set it aside.
- Sizzle butter into a large-sized wok on the burner at around medium heat.
- Cook the mushrooms, olives, scallion, and garlic for around 4-5 minutes.

Place the egg mixture over the vegetables.

Cook for around 4-5 minutes, letting the uncooked portion flow underneath.

Sprinkle the omelet with tuna and cheese and immediately cover the wok.

Take off the burner and set it aside with the cover for around 1-2 minutes.

Cut into serving portions and enjoy.

INGREDIENTS REQUIRED:

- Large-sized eggs – 6
- Whole milk – ¼ C. (60 ml)
- Italian seasoning – 1 tsp.
- Salt and ground black pepper – as desired
- Unsalted butter – 1 tbsp.
- Fresh mushrooms – 3, cut up
- Ripe olives – 2 tbsp. (20 g), pitted and cut up
- Scallion – 1, cut up
- Garlic cloves – 2, minced
- Canned tuna – ¼ C. (145 g), liquid removed and flaked
- Mozzarella cheese – 1 C. (115 g), shredded

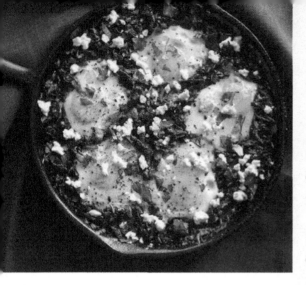

Eggs with Green Veggies

Prep period: 15 mins.
Cook period: 25 mins.
Serves: 4

Per Serving: Calories 275, Fat 20g, Carbs 15.5g, Protein 12.2g

INGREDIENTS REQUIRED:

- Olive oil – ¼ C. (60 ml)
- Brussels sprout – 8 oz. (220 g), trimmed and thinly sliced
- Salt – as desired
- Large-sized onion – ½, finely cut up
- Garlic cloves – 3, minced
- Fresh kale – 8 oz. (220 g), tough ribs removed and cut up
- Fresh baby spinach – 2 C. (60 g)
- Ground coriander – 1 tsp.
- Ground cumin – ½ tsp.
- Red pepper flakes – ½ tsp., crushed
- Water – ½ C. (120 ml)
- Lemon juice – 1 tbsp., freshly squeezed
- Large-sized eggs – 4
- Scallion – 1, cut up
- Feta cheese – ¼ C. (30 g), crumbled

PROCEDURE:

1. Sizzle oil into a 10-inch wok on burner at around medium-high heat.
2. Cook the Brussels sprout and sa for around 5-6 minutes, stirring from time to time.
3. Blend in onions and garlic and immediately turn the heat at around medium.
4. Cook for around 3-4 minutes, stirring frequently.
5. Put in kale, spinach, spices, and water and blend to incorporate.
6. Turn the heat to around mediu low.
7. Cook with the cover for around 8-10 minutes.
8. Put in lemon juice and blend to incorporate.
9. With a spoon, make 4 wells in t greens mixture.
10. Carefully crack 1 egg into each well and sprinkle with a bit of s
11. Cook with the cover for around 4-5 minutes.
12. Take off from the burner and enjoy right away with the garnishing of scallion and feta.

Ham Quiche

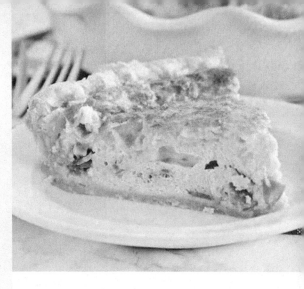

Prep period: 15 mins.
Cook period: 40 mins.
Serves: 6

er Serving: Calories 306, Fat 18.7g,
Carbs 23.4g, Protein 12.2g

PROCEDURE:

For preheating: set your oven at
375 °F (190 °C).
Put the eggshalf-and-half,
garlic, and pepper into a small
basin and whisk to incorporate
thoroughly.
Lay out the pie crust into a 9-inch
quiche pan and sprinkle with feta
cheese.
Place the onion and ham over
cheese, followed by spinach and
red peppers.
Place the egg mixture on top and
sprinkle with mozzarella cheese.
Bake for around 35-40 minutes.
Take off the quiche pan from the
oven and place it onto a cooling
metal rack for around 5 minutes.
Cut into serving portions and
enjoy.

INGREDIENTS REQUIRED:

- Eggs – 5
- Half-and-half – ½ C. (120 g)
- Garlic cloves – 4, cut up
- Ground black pepper – as desired
- Refrigerated pie crust – 1, thawed
- Tomato-basil feta cheese – 1 (4-oz.)
  (110-g) package, crumbled
- Onions – ¼ C. (30 g), finely cut up
- Cooked ham – ½ C. (75 g), cut up
- Fresh baby spinach – 2 C. (60 g),
  roughly cut up
- Roasted red peppers – ½ C. (75 g),
  liquid removed and cut up
- Mozzarella cheese – ½ C. (60 g),
  shredded

Tomato Muffins

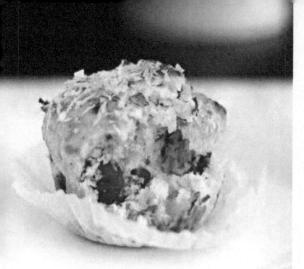

Prep period: 15 mins.

Cook period: 15 mins.

Serves: 6

Per Serving: Calories 323, Fat 17g, Carbs 31.5g, Protein 13.6g

INGREDIENTS REQUIRED:

- Sun-dried tomatoes – 1/3 C. (20 g)
- Whole-wheat flour – 2 C. (260 g)
- Baking powder – 1– ¾ tsp. (7 g)
- Baking soda – ½ tsp. (2 g)
- Salt – ½ tsp. (1¼ g)
- Large-sized egg – 1
- Buttermilk – 1 C. (240 ml)
- Olive oil – ¼ C. (60 ml)
- Soft goat cheese – 4 oz. (110 g), crumbled
- Fresh basil – 2 tbsp. (2½ g), finely cut up

PROCEDURE:

1. For preheating: set your oven at 37 °F (190 °C).
2. Line a 12-hole muffin tin with par liners.
3. Soak the sun-dried tomatoes in a small basin of hot water for aroun 10 minutes.
4. Drain the sun-dried tomatoes and chop them. Set them aside.
5. Put the flour, baking powder, baki soda, and salt into a large-sized basin and blend thoroughly.
6. Put the egg, buttermilk, and oil into another basin and whisk to incorporate them thoroughly.
7. Make a well in the center of the flour mixture.
8. Place the oil mixture into the well and gently stir it with a spatula to incorporate it.
9. Lightly blend in goat cheese, sun-dried tomatoes, and basil.
10. Place the mixture into muffin hol
11. Bake for around 12-15 minutes.
12. Take off the muffin tin from the oven and place it onto a cooling metal rack to cool for around 10 minutes.
13. Carefully turn the muffins onto th metal rack and enjoy moderately hot.

Yogurt Pancakes

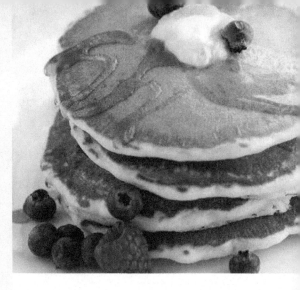

Prep period: 10 mins.
Cook period: 24 mins.
Serves: 6

Per Serving: Calories 203, Fat 4.4g,
Carbs 29.1g, Protein 10g

PROCEDURE:

- Put the oats, flour, flaxseeds, baking soda, and salt into an electric blender and process to incorporate them thoroughly.
- Shift the mixture into a large-sized basin.
- Put in remnant ingredients except the oil and blend to incorporate thoroughly.
- Set it aside for around 20 minutes before cooking.
- Spray an anti-sticking wok with baking spray and sizzle on the burner at around medium heat. Put the desired amount of the mixture into the wok and spread it into an even layer with a spoon.
- Cook for around 2 minutes per side.
- Cook the remnant pancakes in the same manner.
- Enjoy moderately hot.

INGREDIENTS REQUIRED:

- Old-fashioned oats – 1 C. (100 g)
- All-purpose flour – ½ C. (65 g)
- Flaxseeds – 2 tbsp.
- Baking soda – 1 tsp.
- Salt – as desired
- Maple syrup – 2 tbsp.
- Large-sized eggs – 2
- Plain Greek yogurt – 2 C. (500 g)
- Olive oil baking spray

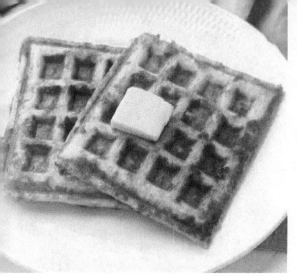

Mozzarella Waffles

Prep period: 10 mins.
Cook period: 10 mins.
Serves: 2

Per Serving: Calories 352, Fat 20.9g
Carbs 23.5g, Protein 22.3g

INGREDIENTS REQUIRED:

- Mozzarella cheese – 2 C. (230 g), shredded
- Almond flour – ¼ C. (25 g)
- Baking powder – 2 tsp.
- Eggs – 4
- Ground cinnamon – 1 tsp.
- White sugar – 2 tbsp.
- Fresh blueberries – 1/3 C. (55 g)
- Olive oil baking spray

PROCEDURE:

1. Put the cheese and remnant ingredients except for blueberries into a basin and whisk to incorporate thoroughly.
2. Lightly blend in blueberries.
3. Preheat the waffle iron and then spray it with baking spray.
4. Place the desired amount of the mixture into the preheated waffle iron.
5. Cook for around 4-5 minutes.
6. Cook the remnant waffle in the same manner.
7. Enjoy moderately hot.

Banana & Date Bread

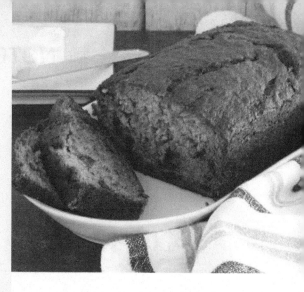

Prep period: 15 mins.
Cook period: 50 mins.
Serves: 12

Per Serving: Calories 227, Fat 8.8g,
Carbs 35.6g, Protein 4.1g

PROCEDURE:

For preheating: set your oven at 325 ºF (165 ºC).
Lightly spray a loaf pan with baking spray.
Put the flour, baking soda, and spices into a basin and blend them to incorporate.
Put the oil and honey into another large-sized basin and whisk thoroughly.
Put in eggs and whisk to incorporate thoroughly.
Put in bananas, milk, yogurt, and vanilla extract and whisk to incorporate thoroughly.
Put in flour mixture and blend until just incorporated.
Lightly blend in dates and walnuts.
Shift the mixture into the loaf pan.
Bake for around 50 minutes.
Take the loaf pan out of the oven and place it onto a cooling metal rack to cool for at least 10-15 minutes.
Carefully turn the bread onto the metal rack to cool thoroughly.
Cut the bread loaf into slices and enjoy.

INGREDIENTS REQUIRED:

- Olive oil baking spray
- All-purpose flour – 1 1/3 C. (180 g)
- Baking soda – 1 tsp.
- Ground cinnamon – ½ tsp.
- Ground cardamom – ½ tsp.
- Ground nutmeg – ½ tsp.
- Olive oil – 1/3 C. (90 ml)
- Honey – ½ C. (150 g)
- Eggs – 2
- Extra-ripe bananas – 3, peel removed and mashed
- Plain Greek yogurt – 2 tbsp. (30 g)
- Whole milk – ¼ C. (60 ml)
- Vanilla extract – 1 tsp.
- Dates – ½ C. (75 g), pitted and cut up
- Walnuts – ½ C. (50 g), cut up

NOTES

APPETIZER & SNACKS RECIPES

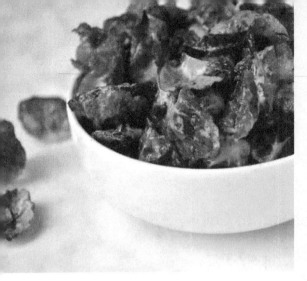

Brussels Sprout Chips

Prep period: 15 mins.
Cook period: 20 mins.
Serves: 3

Per Serving: Calories 100, Fat 6.5g
Carbs 7.6g, Protein 5.4g

INGREDIENTS REQUIRED:

- Olive oil baking spray
- Brussels sprouts – ½ lb. (220 g), thinly sliced
- Parmesan cheese – ¼ C. (30 g), grated and divided
- Olive oil – 1 tbsp. (15 ml)
- Garlic powder – ½ tsp.
- Salt and ground black pepper – as desired

PROCEDURE:

1. For preheating: set your oven a 400 °F (205 °C).
2. Lightly spray a large-sized baking tray with baking spray.
3. Place the Brussels sprout slices 2 tbsp. of Parmesan cheese, oil garlic powder, salt, and pepper into a large-sized basin and tos to incorporate thoroughly.
4. Lay out the Brussels sprout slic onto the baking tray in an ever layer.
5. Bake for around 18-20 minute tossing once halfway through.
6. Take out of the oven and place the Brussels sprouts chips ontc platter.
7. Sprinkle with remnant cheese and enjoy.

Cheese Chips

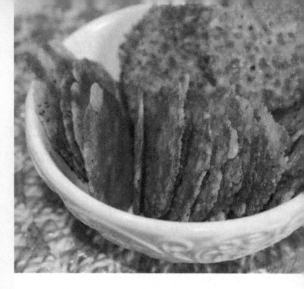

Prep period: 15 mins.

Cook period: 15 mins.

Serves: 8

Per Serving: Calories 94, Fat 7.1g,
Carbs 3.2g, Protein 4.2g

PROCEDURE:

- For preheating: set your oven at 350 °F (175 °C).
- Line a large-sized baking tray with greaseproof paper.
- Put the coconut flour, ¼ C. of mozzarella, Parmesan, butter, and egg into a basin and blend to incorporate thoroughly.
- Set the mixture aside for around 3-5 minutes.
- Make 8 equal-sized balls from the mixture.
- Lay out the balls onto a baking tray about 2 inches apart.
- With your hands, press each ball into a little flat disc
- Sprinkle each disc with the remnant mozzarella, followed by thyme.
- Bake for around 13-15 minutes.
- Take them out of the oven and let them cool thoroughly before enjoying them.

INGREDIENTS REQUIRED:

- Coconut flour – 3 tbsp. (15 g)
- Mozzarella cheese – ½ C. (60 g), grated and divided
- Parmesan cheese – ¼ C. (30 g), grated
- Unsalted butter – 2 tbsp. (30 g), liquefied
- Egg – 1
- Dried thyme – ½ tsp.

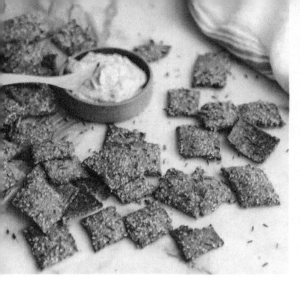

Quinoa Crackers

Prep period: 15 mins.
Cook period: 20 mins.
Serves: 6

Per Serving: Calories 26, Fat 1.6g,
Carbs 2.5g, Protein 1g

INGREDIENTS REQUIRED:

- Water – 3 tbsp. (45 ml)
- Chia seeds – 1 tbsp.
- Sunflower seeds – 3 tbsp.
- Quinoa flour – 1 tbsp.
- Ground turmeric – 1 tsp.
- Ground cinnamon – 1 pinch
- Salt – as desired

PROCEDURE:

1. For preheating: set your oven at 340 °F (170 °C).
2. Line a baking tray with parchment paper.
3. Put the water and chia seeds into a basin and soak them for around 15 minutes.
4. After 15 minutes, put the remaining ingredients in the blender and blend thoroughly.
5. Spread the mixture onto the baking tray.
6. With a pizza cutter, cut the formed mixture into desired shapes.
7. Bake for around 20-25 minutes
8. Take it out of the oven and place it onto a cooling metal rack to cool thoroughly before enjoying it.

Pistachio & Dates Bars

Prep period: 15 mins.
Cook period: 0 mins.
Serves: 8

Per Serving: Calories 175, Fat 7.5g,
Carbs 26.5g, Protein 4.5g

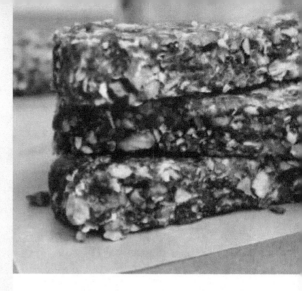

PROCEDURE:

. Put the dates into an electric food processor and process to form a puree.
. Put in pistachios and oats and process to form a crumbly mixture.
. Place the almond butter, applesauce, and vanilla extract in the mixture and process to form a slightly sticky dough.
Place the mixture into an 8x8-inch parchment-lined baking pan.
With the back of a spoon, press down the top surface firmly.
Lay out baking paper on top of the mixture and freeze for around 1 hour before cutting.
Cut into bars and enjoy.

INGREDIENTS REQUIRED:

- Dates – 20, pitted
- Pistachios – 1¼ C. (155 g), roasted
- Old-fashioned rolled oats – 1 C. (1oo g)
- Almond butter – 2 tbsp. (30 g)
- Unsweetened applesauce – ¼ C. (75 g)
- Vanilla extract – 1 tsp.

Almond Brittles

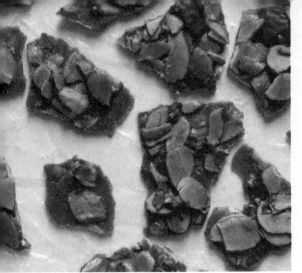

Prep period: 15 mins.

Cook period: 10 mins.

Serves: 8

Per Serving: Calories 123, Fat 11.7g, Carbs 12.7g, Protein 2.6g

INGREDIENTS REQUIRED:

- Almonds – 1 C. (100 g)
- Unsalted butter – ¼ C. (55 g)
- White sugar – ½ C. (100 g)
- Vanilla extract – 2 tsp. (10 ml)
- Salt – ¼ tsp.

PROCEDURE:

1. Line a 9x9-inch cake pan with bakery paper.
2. Put butter, sugar, vanilla, and ¼ tsp. of salt into a non-stick wok on the burner at around mediu heat.
3. Cook for around 2 minutes, stirring all the time.
4. Put in almonds and stir.
5. Cook for around 2-3 minutes, stirring all the time.
6. Take off the wok from the burr and place the mixture into the cake pan.
7. With the back of a spoon, stir t spread the almonds and sprink with salt.
8. Set it aside for around 1 hour.
9. Break into pieces and enjoy.

Stuffed Mushrooms

Prep period: 20 mins.
Cook period: 45 mins.
Serves: 4

r Serving: Calories 362, Fat 24.9g,
Carbs 17.8g, Protein 18.4g

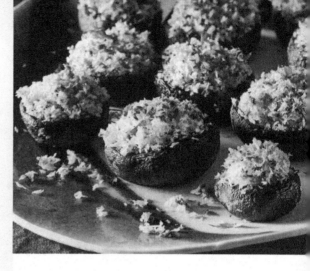

PROCEDURE:

For preheating: set your oven at 350 °F (175 °C).

Spray a baking pan with baking spray.

Drain the clams well, reserving the liquid in a basin.

Put the clams, softened butter, scallion, garlic, oregano, and garlic salt into a basin and blend thoroughly.

Put in the reserved clam juice, breadcrumbs, and egg and blend to incorporate thoroughly.

Put 2 tbsp. of mozzarella and Parmesan cheese and blend thoroughly.

Lay out the mushrooms onto a platter and stuff the cavity of each with a clam mixture.

Lay out the mushrooms into the baking pan and drizzle with melted butter.

Bake for around 35-40 minutes.

Take it out of the oven and sprinkle the mushrooms with remnant mozzarella cheese.

Bake for around 5 minutes.

Garnish with parsley and enjoy.

INGREDIENTS REQUIRED:

- Olive oil baking spray
- Clams – 6 oz. (150 g)
- Unsalted butter – 1 tbsp. (15 g), softened
- Scallion – 1 tbsp., finely cut up
- Garlic cloves – 2, minced
- Dried oregano – 1 tsp.
- Garlic salt – 1 pinch
- Italian breadcrumbs – ½ C. (75 g)
- Egg – 1, whisked
- Mozzarella cheese – 1/3 C. (45 g), grated and divided
- Parmesan cheese – 3 tbsp. (20 g), grated
- Unsalted butter – ¼ C. (55 g) liquefied
- Mushrooms – 8, stems removed
- Fresh parsley – 2 tbsp., cut up

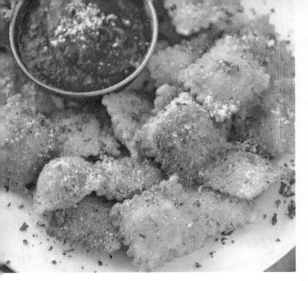

Fried Ravioli

Prep period: 15 mins.
Cook period: 12 mins.
Serves: 8

Per Serving: Calories 416, Fat 29.9
Carbs 33.7g, Protein 8.3g

INGREDIENTS REQUIRED:

- All-purpose flour – 1 C. (130 g)
- Eggs – 2
- Water – ¼ C. (60 ml)
- Breadcrumbs – 1 C. (150 g)
- Italian seasoning – 1 tsp.
- Garlic cloves – 3, minced
- Meat ravioli – 16 oz. (455 g)
- Olive oil – 1-2 C. (240-480 ml)

PROCEDURE:

1. Put the flour into a shallow dis
2. Put the eggs and water into a second shallow dish and whisk thoroughly.
3. Put the breadcrumbs, Italian seasoning, and garlic salt into a third shallow dish and blend to incorporate.
4. Coat each raviolo in flour, then dip it in the egg mixture, and finally coat it with the breadcrumbs mixture.
5. Sizzle oil into a deep wok on th burner at around medium hea
6. Fry the ravioli in 4 batches for around 3 minutes, flipping fro time to time.
7. With a slotted spoon, shift the fried ravioli onto a paper towe lined plate to drain.
8. Enjoy moderately hot.

Bacon-Wrapped Mozzarella Sticks

Prep period: 10 mins.
Cook period: 6 mins.
Serves: 8

er Serving: Calories 453, Fat 42.3g, Carbs 1.4g, Protein 18.7g

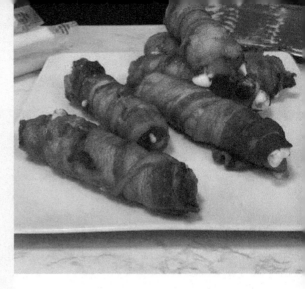

PROCEDURE:

. Wrap a bacon strip around each cheese stick and secure it with a toothpick.
. Sizzle oil into a cast-iron wok on the burner at around medium heat.
. Put mozzarella sticks into 2 batches and fry for around 2-3 minutes.
. With a slotted spoon, shift the mozzarella sticks onto a paper towel-lined plate to drain.
. Set them aside to cool slightly.
. Enjoy moderately hot.

INGREDIENTS REQUIRED:

- Bacon strips – 8
- Mozzarella cheese sticks – 8, frozen overnight
- Olive oil – 1 C. (240 ml)

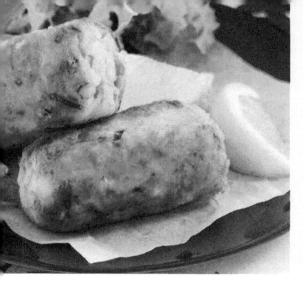

Tuna Croquettes

Prep period: 15 mins.
Cook period: 16 mins.
Serves: 4

Per Serving: Calories 492, Fat 30.2g
Carbs 6.8g, Protein 48.1g

INGREDIENTS REQUIRED:

- Canned white tuna – 24 oz. (680 g), liquid removed
- Mayonnaise – ¼ C. (35 g)
- Large-sized eggs – 4
- Onions – 2 tbsp. (15 g), finely cut up
- Scallion – 1, thinly sliced
- Garlic cloves – 4, minced
- Almond flour – ¾ C. (75 g)
- Salt and ground black pepper – as desired
- Olive oil – ¼ C. (60 ml)

PROCEDURE:

1. Put the tuna, mayonnaise, eggs, onion, scallion, garlic, almond flour, salt, and pepper into a large basin and blend to incorporate thoroughly.
2. Make 8 equal-sized oblong-shaped patties from the mixture
3. Sizzle oil into a large-sized wok on the burner at around medium-high heat.
4. Fry the croquettes in 2 batches for around 2-4 minutes per side
5. With a slotted spoon, shift the croquettes onto a paper towel-lined plate to drain thoroughly.
6. Enjoy moderately hot.

Spinach & Artichoke Dip

Prep period: 15 mins.
Cook period: 20 mins.
Serves: 8

er Serving: Calories 244, Fat 20.3g,
Carbs: 6.1g, Protein 8.2g

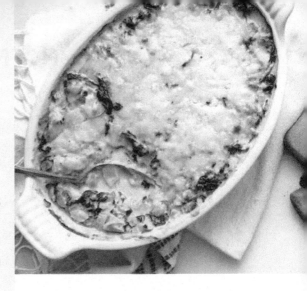

PROCEDURE:

. For preheating: set your oven to 350 ºF (175 ºC).
. Spray a baking pan with baking spray.
. Put the cheeses, sour cream, mayonnaise, garlic, and pepper into a basin and stir to incorporate.
Lightly blend in artichokes and spinach.
Shift the mixture into the baking pan.
Bake for around 20 minutes.
Enjoy right away.

INGREDIENTS REQUIRED:

- Olive oil baking spray
- Cream cheese – 6 oz. (225 g), softened
- Parmesan cheese – 2/3 C. (75g), finely shredded
- Mozzarella cheese – ½ C. (60g), finely shredded
- Sour cream – ¼ C. (60 g)
- Mayonnaise – ¼ C. (35 g)
- Garlic clove – 1, minced
- Ground black pepper – as desired
- Quartered artichoke hearts – 1 (14-oz.) (400-g) can, liquid removed, squeezed, and cut up
- Frozen spinach –6 oz. (150 g), thawed and squeezed

NOTES

VEGETABLE RECIPES

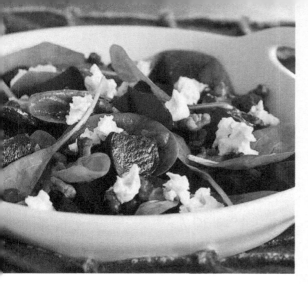

Beet & Walnut Salad

Prep period: 10 mins.
Cook period: 1 hr.
Serves: 4

Per Serving: Calories 378, Fat 28.4
Carbs 22.9g, Protein 11.7g

INGREDIENTS REQUIRED:

For the Salad:
- Medium-sized beets – 6, scrubbed
- Fresh baby spinach – 6 C. (180 g)
- Feta cheese – 4 oz. (110 g), crumbled
- Walnuts – ½ C. (50 g), toasted and cut up

For the Dressing:
- Olive oil – ¼ C. (60 ml)
- Balsamic vinegar – 3 tbsp. (45 ml)
- Maple syrup – 1 tbsp.
- Dijon mustard – 2 tsp.
- Salt and ground black pepper – as desired

PROCEDURE:

1. For preheating: set your oven a 400 °F (205 °C).
2. Wrap each beet in a piece of heavy-duty foil.
3. Lay out the wrapped beets onto baking tray and roast for arou 1 hour.
4. Take out of the oven and unwr the beets.
5. Set them aside to cool thoroughly.
6. Then, peel the beets and cut them into pieces.
7. In the meantime, for the dressing: put the oil and remn ingredients into a basin and whisk to incorporate thoroug
8. Put the beets, spinach, walnut and dressing into a salad dish and toss to incorporate thoroughly.
9. Top with feta and enjoy.

Caprese Salad

Prep period: 10 mins.

Cook period: 0

Serves: 4

Per Serving: Calories 213, Fat 18.2g, Carbs 7.1g, Protein 7.9g

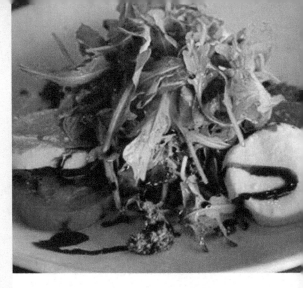

PROCEDURE:

. For the dressing: put the basil and remnant ingredients into an electric blender and process to form a smooth mixture.

. For the salad: put the tomatoes and remnant ingredients into a large-sized salad dish and blend.

. Place the dressing over the salad and toss to incorporate thoroughly.

. Enjoy right away.

INGREDIENTS REQUIRED:

For the Dressing:
- Fresh basil – ½ C. (10 g), cut up
- Garlic cloves – 2, minced
- Olive oil – ¼ C. (60 ml)
- Balsamic vinegar – 2 tbsp. (30 ml)
- Salt and ground black pepper – as desired

For the Salad:
- Medium-sized ripe tomatoes – 4, cut into slices
- Mozzarella cheese – 3 oz. (85 g), cut into slices
- Fresh arugula – 5 C. (100 g)

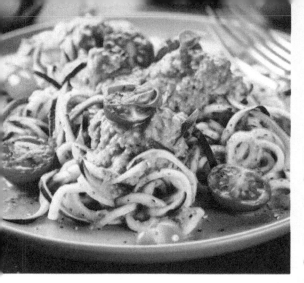

Pesto Zoodles with Tomatoes

Prep period: 20 mins.
Cook period: 7 mins.
Serves: 4

Per Serving: Calories 306, Fat 28.9g
Carbs 16.1g, Protein 3.6g

INGREDIENTS REQUIRED:

- Large-sized zucchinis – 2, spiralized with a blade
- Olive oil – 1 tbsp. (15 ml)
- Fresh kale – 3 C. (155 g), tough ribs removed and cut up
- Fresh basil – ½ C. (10 g)
- Garlic clove – 1, cut up
- Olive oil – ½ C. (120 ml)
- Water – ¼ C. (60 ml)
- Lemon juice – 1 tbsp. (15 ml), freshly squeezed
- Salt and ground black pepper – as desired
- Cherry tomatoes – 1 C. (150 g), halved

PROCEDURE:

1. Put half of the zucchini noodles into a large-sized microwave-safe dish and microwave on high for around 2 minutes.
2. Repeat with the remnant zucchini noodles.
3. Sizzle oil, in the meantime, into a wok on the burner at around medium-high heat.
4. Cook the kale for around 5 minutes.
5. Put the cooked kale and remnant ingredients into an electric food processor and process to form a smooth mixture.
6. Shift the pesto into a large-sized basin.
7. Put in the zucchini noodles and tomatoes and stir to incorporate.

Squash with Fruit

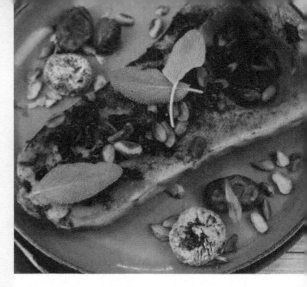

Prep period: 15 mins.

Cook period: 40 mins.

Serves: 4

Per Serving: Calories 227, Fat 5.5g, Carbs 46.4g, Protein 5g

PROCEDURE:

For preheating: set your oven at 375 ºF (190 ºC).

Place the water in the bottom of a large-sized baking pan.

Lay out the squash halves into the baking pan, hollow side up, and drizzle with oil and vinegar. Sprinkle with salt and pepper. Spread the dates, figs, and pistachios on top.

Bake for around 40 minutes. Enjoy right away with the garnishing of pumpkin seeds.

INGREDIENTS REQUIRED:

- Water – ¼ C. (60 ml)
- Medium-sized butternut squash – 1, halved and seeded
- Olive oil – 2 tsp. (10 ml)
- Balsamic vinegar – 2 tsp. (10 ml)
- Salt and ground black pepper – as desired
- Large-sized dates – 4, pitted and cut up
- Fresh figs – 4, cut up
- Pistachios – ¼ C. (30 g), cut up

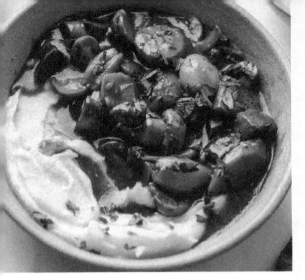

Mushroom Bourguignon

Prep period: 15 mins.

Cook period: 45 mins.

Serves: 4

Per Serving: Calories 144, Fat 7.5g, Carbs 12.5g, Protein 6g

INGREDIENTS REQUIRED:

- Olive oil – 1 tbsp. (15 ml)
- Fresh mushrooms – 10 oz. (280 g), sliced
- Small-sized onion – 1, cut up
- Garlic cloves – 4, minced
- Red wine – ¼ C. (60 ml)
- Tomato paste – 1 tbsp. (20 g)
- Onion powder – 1 tsp.
- Red pepper flakes – ¼ tsp.
- Salt – as desired
- Vegetable broth – 2 C. (480 ml)
- Carrots – 1 C. (150 g), cut up
- Celery stalk – 1, cut up
- Unsalted butter – 1 tbsp.
- All-purpose flour – 1 tbsp.
- Water – 2 tbsp. (30 ml)
- Fresh parsley – ¼ C. (5 g), cut up

PROCEDURE:

1. Sizzle oil into a deep, anti-sticking wok on the burner at around medium heat.
2. Cook the mushrooms, onion and garlic for around 4-5 minutes.
3. Put in wine and stir.
4. Cook for around 1-2 minutes, stirring frequently.
5. Put in the tomato paste, thyme, onion powder, red pepper flakes, and salt.
6. Cook for around 1 minute, stirring frequently.
7. Blend in broth, carrots, and celery and turn the heat at around high.
8. Cook the mixture until boiling.
9. Turn the heat to around medium-low.
10. Cook with the cover for around 3 minutes.
11. In the meantime, for the flour slurry, put the flour and water into a small basin and blend them to dissolve.
12. Put the flour slurry in the pot, stirring all the time.
13. Cook for around 1-2 minutes, constantly stirring.
14. Stir in parsley and enjoy right aw

Eggplant Parmesan

Prep period: 20 mins.

Cook period: 50 mins.

Serves: 8

er Serving: Calories 416, Fat 10.4g, Carbs 49.3g, Protein 14.4g

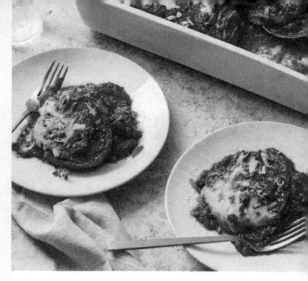

PROCEDURE:

For preheating: set your oven at 350 °F (175 °C).

Generously spray a 13x9-inch baking pan with baking spray.

Place eggs and breadcrumbs, respectively, in 2 different shallow bowls.

Dip the eggplant slices in eggs and then coat with breadcrumbs.

Lay out the eggplant slices onto the baking trays.

Bake for around 15-20 minutes, flipping once halfway through.

Again, set your oven at 350 °F (175 °C).

Put the mushrooms and dried herbs into a small basin and stir.

Put both cheeses into a separate small basin and stir to incorporate.

Place ½ C. of spaghetti sauce in the baking pan and spread.

Place about 1/3 of the mushroom mixture over the sauce, followed by 1/3 of the eggplant slices, ¾ C. of sauce, and 1/3 of the cheese mixture.

Repeat the layers twice.

Bake for around 26-30 minutes.

Enjoy moderately hot.

INGREDIENTS REQUIRED:

- Olive oil baking spray
- Large-sized eggs – 3, whisked
- Panko breadcrumbs – 2½ C. (375 g)
- Medium-sized eggplants – 3, cut into ¼-inch slices
- Sliced mushrooms – 2 (4½-oz.) (230-g) jars, liquid removed
- Dried basil – ½ tsp.
- Dried oregano – ½ tsp.
- Mozzarella cheese – 2 C. (230 g), shredded
- Parmesan cheese – ½ C. (55 g), shredded
- Spaghetti sauce – 2 (14-oz.) (400-g) jars

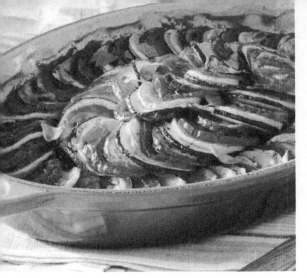

Ratatouille

Prep period: 20 mins.
Cook period: 45 mins.
Serves: 4

Per Serving: Calories 206, Fat 11.4g
Carbs 26.4g, Protein 5.4g

INGREDIENTS REQUIRED:

- Tomato paste – 6 oz. (150 g)
- Olive oil – 3 tbsp. (45 ml), divided
- Medium-sized onion – ½, cut up
- Garlic cloves – 6, minced
- Salt and ground black pepper – as desired
- Water – ¾ C. (180 ml)
- Medium-sized zucchini – 1, sliced into thin circles
- Medium-sized yellow squash – 1, sliced into circles thinly
- Eggplant – 1, sliced into circles thinly
- Medium-sized bell peppers – 2, seeded and sliced into circles thinly
- Fresh thyme – 2 tbsp., minced
- Lemon juice – 1 tbsp. (15 ml), freshly squeezed

PROCEDURE:

1. For preheating: set your oven a 375 ºF (190 ºC).
2. Put the tomato paste, 1 tbsp. of oil, onion, garlic, salt, and pepper into a basin and blend nicely.
3. Place the tomato paste mixture at the bottom of a baking pan and spread it.
4. Arrange alternating vegetable slices, starting at the outer edg of the baking pan and working concentrically towards the center.
5. Drizzle the vegetables with the remnant oil and sprinkle with salt and pepper, followed by th thyme.
6. Arrange a piece of parchment paper over the vegetables.
7. Bake for around 45 minutes.
8. Enjoy right away.

Vegetable Coq Au Vin

Prep period: 15 mins.
Cook period: 30 mins.
Serves: 4

Per Serving: Calories 346, Fat 4.3g,
Carbs 59.5g, Protein 8.3g

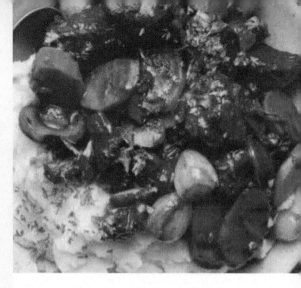

PROCEDURE:

Sizzle oil into a Dutch oven on a burner at around medium heat.
Cook the cut-up onions for around 5 minutes.
Put in the garlic and cook for around 1 minute.
Put in the potatoes, carrots, mushrooms, and pearl onions and blend.
Cook for around 3-4 minutes, stirring frequently.
Put in the flour and tomato paste and blend.
Stir-fry for around 1-2 minutes.
Put in wine and cook for around 3 minutes, stirring frequently.
Put in broth and thyme and stir.
Cook for around 10-15 minutes, stirring from time to time.
Enjoy right away with the decoration of thyme.

INGREDIENTS REQUIRED:

- Olive oil – 1 tbsp. (15 ml)
- Medium-sized onion – 1, cut up
- Garlic cloves – 3, sliced
- Large-sized potatoes – 3, cut into chunky wedges
- Medium-sized carrots – 2, peel removed and sliced
- Fresh mushrooms – 1 C. (125 g), sliced
- Pearl onions – 1 C. (135 g) peel removed
- All-purpose flour – 2 tbsp. (15 g)
- Tomato paste – 1 tbsp. (20 g)
- Red wine – 9 fluid oz. (260 ml)
- Vegetable broth – 1¼ C. (300 ml)
- Fresh thyme – 2 tbsp. (2½ g) cut up

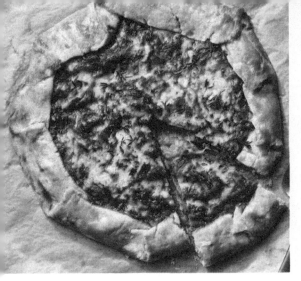

Onion Galette

Prep period: 20 mins.
Cook period: 1 hr. 10 mins.
Serves: 4

Per Serving: Calories 375, Fat 24.9g
Carbs 32.9g, Protein 6.7g

INGREDIENTS REQUIRED:

For the Dough:
- All-purpose flour – ½ C. (65 g) plus more for dusting
- Whole-wheat flour – ½ C. (65 g)
- Salt – ½ tsp.
- Chilled butter – 1/3 C. (85 g), cut into pieces
- Ice cold water – 5 tbsp. (75 ml)

For the Filling:
- Unsalted butter – 2 tbsp. (30 g)
- Medium-sized onions – 3, thinly sliced
- Dried thyme – 1 tsp.
- Salt and ground black pepper – as desired
- Egg – 1, whisked

PROCEDURE:

1. For the dough: put the flour and salt into a basin and blend thoroughly.
2. With a pastry cutter, cut in the butter to form a coarse meal-li mixture.
3. Slowly put in water and blend until just incorporated.
4. With your hands, gently kneac until the dough comes togethe
5. With your hands, flatten the dough into a disk.
6. With plastic wrap, cover the dough disk and put it into you fridge for around 1 hour.
7. For the filling, sizzle butter int a wok on the burner at mediu high heat.
8. Cook the onions and thyme fc around 10 minutes, stirring fr time to time.
9. Turn the heat to around low.
10. Cook for around 10-15 minut stirring from time to time.
11. Blend in salt and pepper and take off the burner. Set it asid cool.

NOTES

PROCEDURE:

12. For preheating: set your oven at 375 ºF (190 ºC).
13. Lay out a pizza stone on the bottom rack of the oven.
14. Line a baking tray with baking paper.
15. Unwrap the dough and place it onto a lightly floured surface.
16. With a rolling pin, roll the dough into a 12-inch circle.
17. Lay out the dough circle onto the baking tray.
18. Place the onions on the dough circle, leaving about a 1½-inch border.
19. Fold the edge of the dough over the filling and then brush the edges with the whisked egg.
20. Place the baking tray over the pizza stone and bake for around 40 minutes.
21. Now place the baking tray onto the top rack of the oven and bake for around 5 minutes.
22. Take the galette out of the oven and place it onto a rack to cool slightly.
23. Enjoy moderately hot.

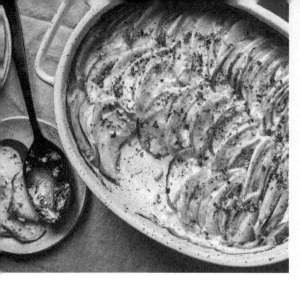

Potato Gratin

Prep period: 15 mins.
Cook period: 55 mins.
Serves: 6

Per Serving: Calories 235, Fat 9.1g,
Carbs 33.7g, Protein 6.2g

INGREDIENTS REQUIRED:

- Olive oil – 2 tbsp. (30 ml)
- Medium-sized onion – 1, thinly sliced
- Garlic cloves – 4, finely cut up
- Whole milk – 1½ C. (350 ml)
- Heavy cream – 1 C. (250 g)
- Apple cider vinegar – 1 tsp. (5 ml)
- Parmesan cheese – ¼ C. (30 g)
- Fresh rosemary sprig – 1, finely cut up
- Ground nutmeg – ¼ tsp.
- Salt and ground black pepper – as desired
- Yellow flesh potatoes – 2¼ lb. (900 g), peel removed and cut into ¼-inch thick slices

PROCEDURE:

1. For preheating: set your oven at 3⁵ ºF (200 ºC).
2. Sizzle oil into a large-sized pot on a burner at around medium-high heat.
3. Cook the onion for around 3-5 minutes.
4. Put in garlic and cook for around minutes.
5. Put in the remnant ingredients except for potatoes and stir.
6. Cook the mixture until boiling.
7. Cook for around 3 minutes, stirri from time to time.
8. Take off from the burner and set i aside.
9. Put the potato slices in the pot of cream mixture and gently stir to incorporate.
10. Shift the potato slices into a bakir pan and spread in an even layer.
11. With a piece of heavy-duty foil, cover the baking pan and gently press down onto the potatoes.
12. Bake for around 20 minutes.
13. Take off the foil piece and bake fc around 20 minutes.
14. Enjoy right away.

SOUP RECIPES

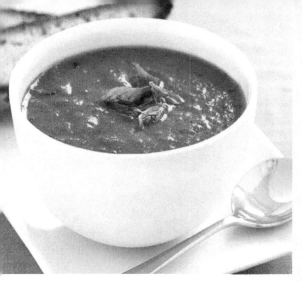

Tomato & Basil Soup

Prep period: 10 mins.
Cook period: 15 mins.
Serves: 4

Per Serving: Calories 108, Fat 3g,
Carbs 19.5g, Protein 4.3g

INGREDIENTS REQUIRED:

- Olive oil – 2 tsp. (10 ml)
- Medium-sized onion – 1, cut up
- Garlic cloves – 3, minced
- Fresh plum tomatoes – 7 C. cut up (1250 g)
- Fresh basil – ½ C. (10 g), cut up
- Salt and ground black pepper – as desired
- Cayenne pepper powder – ¼ tsp.

PROCEDURE:

1. Sizzle oil into a large-sized soup pot on a burner at around medium heat.
2. Cook the onion and garlic for around 5-6 minutes.
3. Put in tomatoes and stir.
4. Cook for around 6-8 minutes, crushing with the back of the spoon from time to time.
5. Blend in basil, salt, and cayenn powder, and take off from the burner.
6. With a hand blender, puree the soup mixture to form a smooth mixture.
7. Enjoy right away.

Zucchini Soup

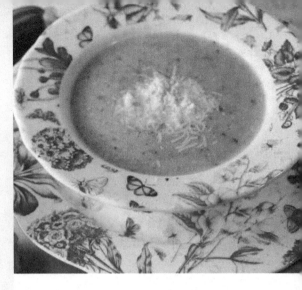

Prep period: 15 mins.

Cook period: 35 mins.

Serves: 6

Per Serving: Calories 115, Fat 6g, Carbs 9.8g, Protein 6.6g

PROCEDURE:

. Sizzle butter into a large-sized soup pot on a burner at around medium heat.

. Cook the onions for around 5-6 minutes.

. Put in garlic and cook for around 1 minute.

. Put in zucchini cubes and blend. Cook for around 5 minutes.

. Blend in thyme, broth, salt, and pepper, and turn the heat to high. Cook the mixture until boiling. Turn the heat to low.

Cook with the cover for around 15-20 minutes.

. Take off the burner and discard the thyme sprigs.

Set the pot aside to cool slightly.

. Put the soup into a large, electric blender in batches and process to form a smooth mixture. Return the soup to the same pot on the burner at around medium heat.

Cook for around 2-3 minutes. Blend in lemon juice and enjoy right away with the garnishing of cheese and lemon peel.

INGREDIENTS REQUIRED:

- Unsalted butter – 2 tbsp. (30 g)
- Medium-sized onions – 2, cut up
- Garlic cloves – 6, minced
- Zucchinis – 6 C. (700 g), cubed
- Fresh thyme sprigs – 4
- Vegetable broth – 4 C. (960 ml)
- Salt and ground black pepper – as desired
- Lemon juice – 2 tbsp. (30 ml), freshly squeezed
- Parmesan cheese – ¼ C. (30 g), shredded
- Lemon peel – 2 tsp., finely grated

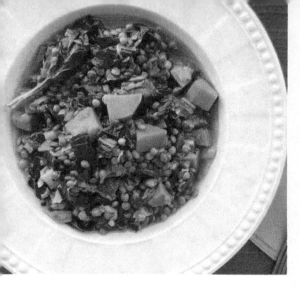

Lentil & Veggie Soup

Prep period: 15 mins.
Cook period: 45 mins.
Serves: 4

Per Serving: Calories 455, Fat 4.5g, Carbs 89.6g, Protein 17.2g

INGREDIENTS REQUIRED:

- Olive oil – 1 tbsp. (15 ml)
- Medium-sized carrots – 2, peel removed and cut up
- Onions – 1 C. (120 g), cut up
- Garlic cloves – 4, minced
- Fresh ginger – 1 tsp., finely cut up
- Sweet potatoes – 3 C. (400 g), peel removed and cubed
- Vegetable broth – 5-6 C. (1200-1450 ml)
- Green lentils – 1 C. (210 g), rinsed and liquid removed
- Fresh baby spinach – 4 C. (120 g)
- Lemon juice – 2 tbsp. (30 ml), freshly squeezed
- Salt and ground black pepper – as desired

PROCEDURE:

1. Sizzle oil into a large-sized pot on a burner at around medium heat.
2. Cook the carrots, onion, garlic, and ginger for around 3-5 minutes.
3. Put in sweet potatoes and blend
4. Cook for around 3-5 minutes, stirring from time to time.
5. Blend in lentils and broth and turn the heat to medium-high.
6. Cook the mixture until boiling
7. Turn the heat to around low.
8. Cook for around 20-25 minute
9. Blend in spinach and blend.
10. Cook for around 3-5 minutes.
11. Put in lemon juice, salt, and pepper, and take off the burner
12. Enjoy right away.

Tortellini & Spinach Soup

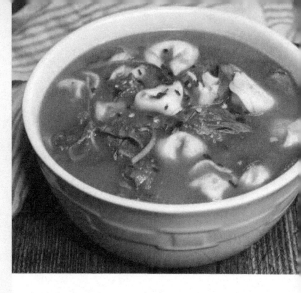

Prep period: 15 mins.
Cook period: 25 mins.
Serves: 8

Per Serving: Calories 192, Fat 7.1g,
Carbs 23.9g, Protein 9.3g

PROCEDURE:

Sizzle oil into a large-sized Dutch oven on the burner at around medium heat.
Cook the onions for around 3-4 minutes, stirring all the time.
Put in garlic and cook for around 1 minute, stirring all the time.
Blend in broth and Italian seasoning and turn the heat at around medium-high.
Cook the mixture until boiling.
Turn the heat to around medium.
Cook for around 5 minutes.
In the meantime, cook tortellini according to the package's directions
Drain the tortellini.
Put the cooked tortellini and tomatoes into the soup mixture and blend.
Cook for around 5 minutes.
Put in spinach and blend.
Cook for around 3-5 minutes.
Add salt and pepper, and enjoy right away.

INGREDIENTS REQUIRED:

- Olive oil – 2 tbsp. (30 ml)
- Medium-sized onion – 1, peel removed and finely cut up
- Garlic cloves – 3, peel removed and minced
- Chicken broth – 6-7 C. (1450-1650 ml)
- Italian seasoning – 2 tsp.
- Refrigerated cheese tortellini – 1 (9-oz.) (250-g) package
- Crushed tomatoes – 2 (14-oz.) (400-g) cans (with juices)
- Fresh spinach – 8 oz. (220 g), cut up
- Salt and ground black pepper – as desired

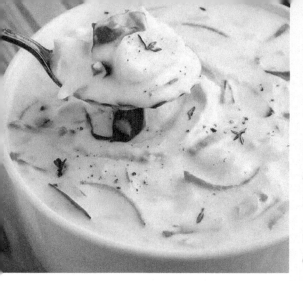

Chicken & Gnocchi Soup

Prep period: 15 mins.
Cook period: 20 mins.
Serves: 8

Per Serving: Calories 380, Fat 23.1g
Carbs 29.4g, Protein 13.6g

INGREDIENTS REQUIRED:

- Unsalted butter – ¼ C. (55 g)
- Olive oil – 1 tbsp. (15 ml)
- Onions – 1 C. (120 g), finely cut up
- Celery stalk – 1, finely cut up
- Garlic cloves – 2, minced
- All-purpose flour – ¼ C. (35 g)
- Half-and-half – 4 C. (950 g)
- Chicken broth – 3½ C. (850 ml)
- Ready-to-use gnocchi – 1 (16-oz.) (455-g) package
- Cooked chicken – 1 C. (140 g), cut up
- Fresh spinach – 1 C. (30 g), cut up
- Carrots – 1 C. (150 g), peel removed and shredded finely
- Dried parsley flakes – ½ tsp. (1 g)
- Dried thyme – ½ tsp.
- Ground nutmeg – ¼ tsp.
- Salt – as desired

PROCEDURE:

1. Sizzle butter and oil into a large sized soup pot on a burner at medium heat.
2. Cook the onion, celery, and garlic for 5-6 minutes, stirring from time to time.
3. Put in the flour and blend.
4. Cook for around 1 minute.
5. Put in half-and-half and whisk to incorporate thoroughly.
6. Cook until thickened, stirring the time.
7. Put in broth and blend.
8. Cook until thickened.
9. Put in gnocchi, chicken, spinac carrots, dried herbs, nutmeg, and salt, and blend.
10. Cook for around 3-5 minutes, stirring from time to time.
11. Enjoy right away.

Meatballs & Orzo Soup

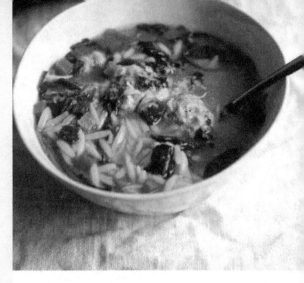

Prep period: 20 mins.
Cook period: 1 hr.
Serves: 6

er Serving: Calories 360, Fat 15.8g,
Carbs 24.2g, Protein 30.3g

PROCEDURE:

For the meatballs: put the ground turkey and remnant ingredients, except for oil, into a large basin and blend to incorporate thoroughly.
Make small-sized balls from the mixture.
Sizzle oil into a large-sized, anti-sticking wok on the burner at around medium-high heat.
Cook the meatballs in 2 batches for around 4 minutes, flipping from time to time.
With a slotted spoon, shift the meatballs onto a paper towel-lined plate.
For the soup: sizzle oil into a large soup pot on a burner at around medium heat.
Cook the onions, carrots, and celery for around 6-8 minutes, stirring frequently.
Put in garlic and cook for around 1 minute.
Blend in broth, salt, and pepper, and turn the heat to high.
Cook the mixture until boiling.
Put in pasta and meatballs and stir.
Again, cook the mixture until boiling.
Turn the heat to around medium-low.
Cook with the cover on for around 10 minutes, stirring from time to time.
Put in spinach and stir.
Cook for around 2-3 minutes.
Enjoy right away.

INGREDIENTS REQUIRED:

For the Meatballs:
- Lean ground turkey – 1 lb. (455 g)
- Large-sized egg – 1
- Parmesan cheese – ½ C. (55 g), finely shredded
- Breadcrumbs – ½ C. (75 g)
- Fresh parsley – ¼ C. (5 g), cut up
- Salt and ground black pepper – as desired
- Olive oil – 1 tbsp. (15 ml)

For the Soup:
- Olive oil – 1 tbsp. (15 ml)
- Onions – 1¼ C. (150 g), cut up
- Carrots – 1¼ C. (190 g), peel removed and cut up
- Celery stalk – 1, cut up
- Garlic cloves – 4, minced
- Chicken broth – 7 C. (1650 ml)
- Salt and ground black pepper – as desired
- Orzo pasta – 1 C. (170 g)
- Fresh spinach – 6 oz. (150 g), cut up

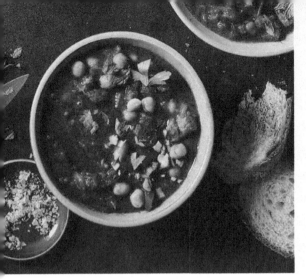

Lamb & Chickpea Soup

Prep period: 15 mins.

Cook period: 2¼ hrs.

Serves: 8

Per Serving: Calories 537, Fat 15g, Carbs 49.9g, Protein 51g

INGREDIENTS REQUIRED:

- Boneless lamb shoulder – 2 lb. (900 g), cubed
- Salt and ground black pepper – as desired
- Olive oil – 2 tbsp. (30 ml)
- Medium-sized onion – 1, cut up
- Garlic cloves – 2, cut up
- Tomato paste – 2 tbsp. (40 g)
- Sweet paprika – 2 tsp.
- Ground cumin – ½ tsp.
- Ground cloves – ½ tsp.
- Diced tomatoes – 2 (14-oz.) (400-g) cans (with juice)
- Chicken broth – 6 C. (1450 ml)
- Chickpeas – 4 (14-oz.) (400-g) cans, liquid removed
- Fresh parsley – ¼ C. (5 g), cut up

PROCEDURE:

1. Rub the lamb cubes with salt and pepper.
2. Sizzle oil into a large-sized pot on burner at medium-high heat.
3. Sear the lamb cubes in 2 batches f around 4-5 minutes.
4. With a slotted spoon, shift the lam cubes into a basin.
5. Put the onion and garlic In the same pot on the burner at mediu heat.
6. Cook for around 3-4 minutes.
7. Put in cooked lamb, tomato paste and spices and blend.
8. Cook for around 1 minute.
9. Blend in the tomatoes and broth and turn the heat at around high
10. Cook the mixture until boiling.
11. Turn the heat to low.
12. Cook with the cover for 1 hour.
13. Put in chickpeas and blend.
14. Cook with the cover for around minutes.
15. Take off the lid and cook for arou 30 minutes more.
16. Stir in salt and pepper and take c the pot of soup from the burner.
17. Enjoy right away with the garnishing of parsley.

Ham & Split Peas Soup

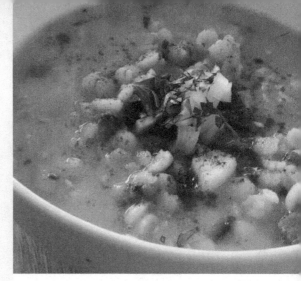

Prep period: 10 mins.
Cook period: 1½ hrs.
Serves: 8

Per Serving: Calories 336, Fat 9.1g,
Carbs 38g, Protein 26g

PROCEDURE:

Sizzle butter into a large-sized soup pot on a burner at medium-low heat.
Cook the celery, onions, and garlic for around 9-10 minutes, stirring frequently.
Blend in ham, split peas, bay leaf, broth, and water, and turn the heat to high.
Cook the mixture until boiling. Turn the heat to low.
Cook with the cover on for around 1½ hours, stirring from time to time.
Stir in salt and pepper, and enjoy right away.

INGREDIENTS REQUIRED:

- Unsalted butter – 2 tbsp. (30 g)
- Celery stalks – 2, cut up
- Medium-sized onion – ½, cut up
- Garlic cloves – 3, sliced
- Ham – 1 lb. (455 g), cut up
- Dried split peas – 1 lb. (455 g), rinsed
- Bay leaf – 1
- Chicken broth – 4 C. (960 ml)
- Water – 2½ C. (600 ml)
- Salt and ground black pepper – as desired

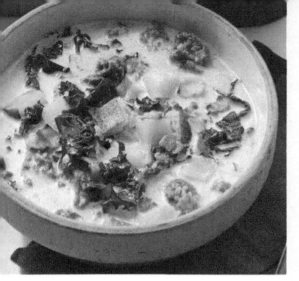

Sausage, Potato & Kale Soup

Prep period: 15 mins.
Cook period: 40 mins.
Serves: 6

Per Serving: Calories 362, Fat 29.4g
Carbs 6.2g, Protein 18.1g

INGREDIENTS REQUIRED:

- Mild Italian sausage – 1 lb. (455 g)
- Medium-sized onion – 1, cut up
- Garlic cloves – 3, peel removed and minced
- Potatoes – 1½ lb. (680 g), scrubbed and cubed
- Chicken broth – 2 C. (480 ml)
- Water – 4 C. (960 ml)
- Red pepper flakes – ½ tsp.
- Salt and ground black pepper – as desired
- Fresh kale – 3 C. (165 g), tough ribs removed and cut up
- Heavy cream – 1 C. (240 g)

PROCEDURE:

1. Sizzle a large-sized soup pot on the burner at medium-high hea
2. Cook the sausage for around 6-8 minutes, crumbling with a wooden spoon.
3. Put in onions and garlic and blend.
4. Cook for around 3-4 minutes.
5. Put in potato, broth, water, red pepper flakes, salt, and pepper and stir.
6. Cook the mixture until boiling
7. Turn the heat to medium.
8. Cook for around 20-25 minute
9. Stir in kale and turn the heat to low.
10. Cook for 2-3 minutes.
11. Put in the cream and stir.
12. Cook for around 2-3 minutes, stirring all the time.
13. Enjoy right away.

Halibut & Quinoa Soup

Prep period: 15 mins.

Cook period: 1 hr.

Serves: 6

Per Serving: Calories 362, Fat 14.7g, Carbs 30.8g, Protein 27.9g

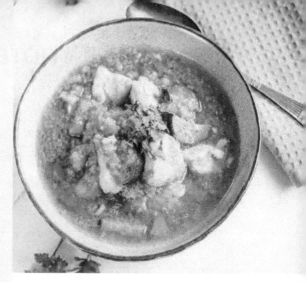

PROCEDURE:

Put the onions, celery, carrot, potato garlic, quinoa, and broth into a large-sized soup pot on a burner at high heat.

Cook the mixture until boiling.

Turn the heat to around low.

Cook with the cover on for around 45 minutes.

Lay out the halibut fillets over the soup mixture.

Cook with the cover on for around 10 minutes.

Stir in salt and pepper, and enjoy right away.

INGREDIENTS REQUIRED:

- Onions – 2 C. (240 g), peel removed and cut up
- Celery stalk – 1, trimmed and cut up
- Carrots – 1 C. (150 g), peel removed and cut up
- Potatoes – 2 C. (240 g), peel removed and cut up
- Garlic cloves – 2, peel removed and cut up
- Quinoa – 1 C. (190 g), rinsed
- Chicken broth – 6 C.
- Halibut fillets – 1 lb. (455 g), cubed
- Salt and ground black pepper – as desired
- Fresh parsley – ¼ C. (5 g), cut up

NOTES

PIZZA & PASTA RECIPES

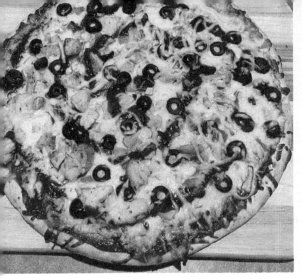

Chicken & Olives Pizza

Prep period: 10 mins.
Cook period: 12 mins.
Serves: 4

Per Serving: Calories 356, Fat 10.7
Carbs 45.6g, Protein 19g

INGREDIENTS REQUIRED:

- Italian cheese-flavored pizza crust – 1 (10-oz.) (280 g)
- Pasta sauce – 1 1/3 C. (410 g)
- Red pepper flakes – ¼ tsp., crushed
- Cooked chicken – 4 oz. (110 g)
- Olives – ¼ C. (45 g), pitted and sliced
- Onions – 2 tbsp. (15 g), cut up
- Mozzarella cheese – ¾ C. (85 g), shredded

PROCEDURE:

1. For preheating: set your oven a 450 °F (230 °C).
2. Lay out the pizza crust onto a baking tray.
3. Spread pasta sauce over the pi: crust, leaving about a 1-inch border.
4. Sprinkle with red pepper flake
5. Place chicken pieces, olives, an onion on top and sprinkle wit cheese.
6. Bake for around 12 minutes.
7. Take it out of the oven and set the pizza aside for around 5 minutes.
8. Cut into serving portions and enjoy.

Mushroom Pizza

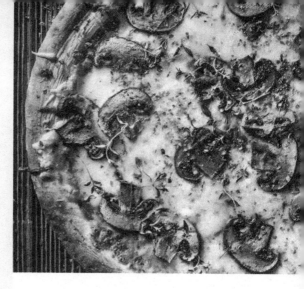

Prep period: 15 mins.
Cook period: 17 mins.
Serves: 6

Per Serving: Calories 210, Fat 5.7g,
Carbs 30.8g, Protein 9.9g

PROCEDURE:

For preheating: set your oven at 450 °F (230 °C).

Spray a large-sized anti-sticking wok with baking spray and sizzle on the burner at medium-high heat.

Cook the mushrooms for around 5 minutes.

Take off from burner.

Put the ricotta and Parmesan cheeses into a basin and blend to incorporate.

Lay out the pizza crust onto a baking tray.

Spread the pasta sauce over the crust, leaving about 1-inch border.

Place the cheese mixture over the sauce and top with mushrooms and mozzarella cheese.

Bake for around 12 minutes.

Take it out of the oven and top with basil.

Set the pizza aside for around 5 minutes.

Cut into serving portions and enjoy.

INGREDIENTS REQUIRED:

- Olive oil baking spray
- Pre-sliced mushrooms – 1 (8-oz.) (225-g) package
- Ricotta cheese – ½ C. (110 g), crumbled
- Parmesan cheese – ¼ C. (30 g), shredded
- Italian cheese-flavored pizza crust – 1 (10-oz.) (285 g)
- Chunky vegetable pasta sauce – 1 C. (300 g)
- Mozzarella cheese – ½ C. (50 g), shredded
- Fresh basil – 2 tbsp., thinly sliced

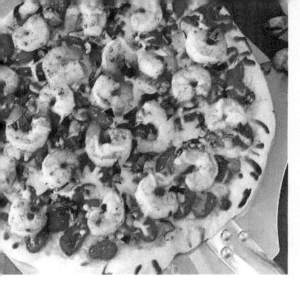

Shrimp & Tomato Pita Pizza

Prep period: 15 mins.
Cook period: 7 mins.
Serves: 6

Per Serving: Calories 373, Fat 14.6g
Carbs 30.1g, Protein 22.8g

INGREDIENTS REQUIRED:

- Cooked small-sized shrimp – ½ lb. (225 g)
- Olive oil – 2 tbsp. (30 ml), divided
- Garlic cloves – 2, minced
- Fresh basil – 2 tbsp., cut up
- Ground black pepper – ½ tsp.
- Onion-flavored pita bread – 4
- Feta cheese – 4 oz. (110 g), crumbled
- Cherry tomatoes – 1 C. (150 g), quartered
- Mozzarella cheese – 1 C. (115 g), shredded

PROCEDURE:

1. For preheating: set your oven at 500 °F (260 °C).
2. Put the shrimp, 1 tbsp. of oil, garlic, herbs, and pepper into a basin and toss it to coat it thoroughly.
3. Set it aside for around 10 minutes.
4. Lay out the pita bread onto a baking tray.
5. Brush the top of each pita with remnant oil and sprinkle with feta and olives.
6. Top each bread with shrimp mixture and sprinkle with mozzarella.
7. Bake for around 6-7 minutes.
8. Take it out of the oven and enjoy it right away.

Orzo & Veggie Salad

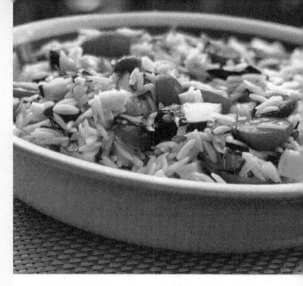

Prep period: 15 mins.
Cook period: 10 mins.
Serves: 4

er Serving: Calories 340, Fat 25.1g,
Carbs 25.2g, Protein 7.9g

PROCEDURE:

For the salad: cook the orzo in a large-sized pot of salted boiling water for around 8-10 minutes. Drain the orzo and rinse under cold running water.
Set it aside to cool.
Put the pasta and remnant ingredients into a large-sized salad dish and blend.
For the dressing: put the oil and remnant ingredients into a small-sized basin and whisk to incorporate thoroughly.
Place the dressing over the salad and toss to incorporate thoroughly.
Put into your fridge to chill thoroughly before enjoying.

INGREDIENTS REQUIRED:

For the Salad
• Uncooked whole-wheat orzo pasta – ½ C. (85 g)
• Cherry tomatoes – 1 C. (150 g), halved
• Black olives – 1 C. (180 g), pitted and sliced
• Cucumber – 1 C. (120 g), cut up
• Onions – ¼ C. (30 g), cut up
• Capers – 1 tbsp. (8 g), liquid removed
For the Dressing
• Olive oil – 1/3 C. (90 ml)
• Lemon juice – 4 tsp. (20 ml) freshly squeezed
• Fresh parsley – 2 tbsp., minced
• Lemon zest – 2 tsp., grated
• Salt and ground black pepper – as desired

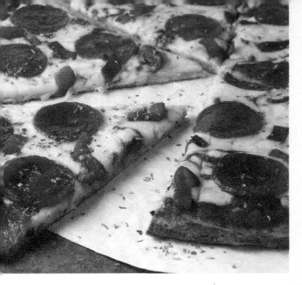

Pepperoni Pizza

Prep period: 10 mins.
Cook period: 12 mins.
Serves: 6

Per Serving: Calories 243, Fat 10.1g
Carbs 28.5g, Protein 9.6g

INGREDIENTS REQUIRED:

- Tomato-and-basil pasta sauce – 1 C. (300 g)
- Prebaked whole-wheat thin Italian pizza crust – 1 (10-oz.) (285-g) package
- Turkey pepperoni slices – ¼ C. (35 g)
- Mozzarella cheese – 1½ C. (170 g), shredded

PROCEDURE:

1. For preheating: set your oven a 450 ºF (230 ºC).
2. Place the pasta sauce over the crust, leaving about 1-inch border.
3. Top with half of the pepperoni slices and sprinkle with cheese.
4. Top with remnant pepperoni slices.
5. Lay out the pizza directly on th oven rack.
6. Bake for around 11-12 minute:
7. Take it out of the oven and set the pizza aside for around 5 minutes.
8. Cut into serving portions and enjoy.

Spinach & Olives Pita Pizza

Prep period: 10 mins.
Cook period: 5 mins.
Serves: 4

er Serving: Calories 344, Fat 12.8g,
Carbs 43.9g, Protein 14.4g

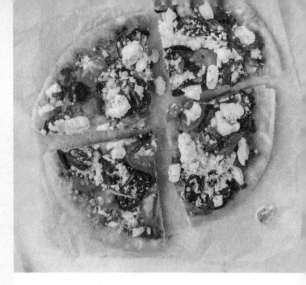

PROCEDURE:

For preheating: set your oven at 400 °F (205 °C).
Place the pita breads in an ungreased 15½ x 10½-inch flat baking pan.
Spread hummus onto each pita bread and sprinkle with cheese.
Bake for around 8-10 minutes.
Take out of the oven and top each pizza with onion, spinach, tomato, and olives.
Enjoy right away.

INGREDIENTS REQUIRED:

- Pita breads – 4
- Roasted garlic-flavored hummus – ½ C. (110 g)
- Feta cheese – 1 C. (110 g), crumbled
- Small-sized onion – 1, sliced
- Fresh spinach – 2 C. (60 g), shredded
- Large-sized tomato – 1, seeded and cut up
- Kalamata olives – ¼ C. (45 g), pitted and sliced

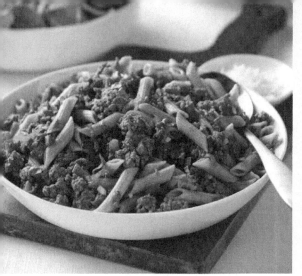

Pasta with Beef & Tomatoes

Prep period: 15 mins.
Cook period: 30 mins.
Serves: 6

Per Serving: Calories 377, Fat 9.3g
Carbs 40.5g, Protein 33.3g

INGREDIENTS REQUIRED:

- Lean ground beef – 1 lb. (455 g)
- Olive oil – 1 tbsp. (15 ml)
- Medium-sized onion – 1, cut up
- Garlic cloves – 3, minced
- Tomatoes – 3 C. (600 g), cut up
- Chicken broth – 1 C. (250 ml)
- Dried basil – ½ tsp.
- Dried parsley – ½ tsp.
- Dried oregano – ½ tsp.
- Ground black pepper – as desired
- Whole-wheat pasta – 1½ C. (300 g)

PROCEDURE:

1. Sizzle a large-sized wok on the burner at medium-high heat.
2. Cook the beef for around 6-8 minutes, stirring from time to time.
3. Take off the wok of beef from th burner and drain the grease.
4. Sizzle oil into a large-sized pot c a burner at medium-high heat.
5. Cook the onion for around 5 minutes.
6. Blend in the garlic and cook for around 1 minute.
7. Put in tomatoes, broth, dried herbs, and pepper and blend.
8. Cook the mixture until boiling.
9. Turn the heat to around low.
10. Cook for around 10 minutes.
11. In the meantime, cook the past in a pot of lightly salted boiling water for 8-10 minutes.
12. Drain the pasta.
13. Put the beef in the pot of the tomato mixture and blend.
14. Cook for around 10 minutes.
15. Put in pasta and toss to incorporate.
16. Enjoy right away.

Pasta with Shrimp & Spinach

Prep period: 15 mins.
Cook period: 12 mins.
Serves: 4

Per Serving: Calories 343, Fat 6.8g,
Carbs 36.9g, Protein 34.5g

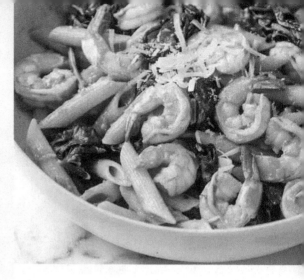

PROCEDURE:

Cook the pasta in a large-sized pot of lightly salted boiling water for around 10 minutes.
In the meantime, sizzle oil into a large-sized wok on the burner at medium heat.
Cook the shrimp for around 2 minutes.
Put in the spinach and garlic and blend.
Cook for around 2 minutes.
Put in pasta, basil, salt, and pepper and toss to incorporate.
Enjoy right away with a sprinkling of cheese.

INGREDIENTS REQUIRED:

- Whole-wheat pasta – 8 oz. (225 g)
- Olive oil – 2 tbsp. (30 ml)
- Shrimp – 12 oz. (340 g), peeled and deveined
- Frozen spinach – 1 (10-oz.) (280-g) package, thawed
- Garlic cloves – 3, cut up
- Dried basil – 2 tsp., crushed
- Salt and ground black pepper – as desired
- Parmesan cheese – ¼ C. (30 g), grated

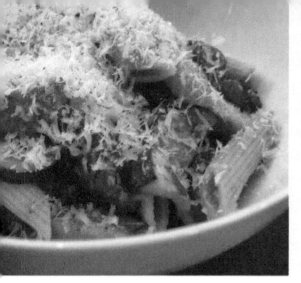

Pasta with Zucchini & Tomatoes

Prep period: 15 mins.
Cook period: 10 mins.
Serves: 6

Per Serving: Calories 296, Fat 10.1g
Carbs 42.2g, Protein 11.1g

INGREDIENTS REQUIRED:

- Whole-wheat penne pasta – 10 oz. (280 g)
- Olive oil – 3 tbsp. (45 ml), divided
- Zucchinis – 1 lb. (455 g), cut into bite-sized pieces
- Cherry tomatoes – 1 lb. (455 g), halved
- Garlic cloves – 6, minced
- Fresh parsley – ½ C. (10 g), finely cut up
- Salt and ground black pepper – as desired
- Parmesan cheese – ½ C. (55 g), shredded

PROCEDURE:

1. Cook the pasta in a large pot of lightly salted boiling water for 10 minutes.
2. Drain the pasta thoroughly.
3. In the meantime, sizzle 1 tbsp. of oil into a large-sized anti-sticking wok on the burner at around medium-high heat.
4. Cook the zucchini for around 5 minutes, stirring from time to time.
5. With a slotted spoon, place the zucchini into a basin and set it aside.
6. Sizzle 1 tbsp of oil in the same wok.
7. Cook the tomatoes for around 3 minutes, stirring from time to time.
8. Put in garlic and cook for around 1 minute, stirring frequently.
9. Take off the wok of tomato mixture from the burner and blend in cooked pasta, zucchini, parsley, remnant oil, salt and pepper.
10. Top with Parmesan and enjoy right away.

Sausage Lasagna

Prep period: 20 mins.
Cook period: 1 hr. 40 mins.
Serves: 8

er Serving: Calories 455, Fat 23.7g,
Carbs 33.4g, Protein 27.4g

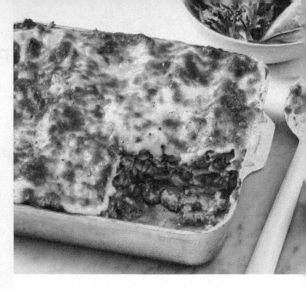

PROCEDURE:

Sizzle a 10-inch wok on the burner at around medium heat.
Cook the sausage, onion, and garlic for around 6-8 minutes, stirring from time to time.
Drain the grease from the wok.
Put in tomatoes and tomato sauce for 2 tbsp. of parsley and sugar and blend.
Cook the mixture until boiling, stirring from time to time.
Turn the heat to around low.
Cook for around 45 minutes.
For preheating: set your oven at 350 °F (175 °C).
In the meantime, cook the noodles as directed on the package.
Drain the noodles.
Put the ricotta cheese, ¼ C. of Parmesan cheese, remnant parsley, and oregano into a medium basin and blend thoroughly.
Put about 1 C. of the sauce in the bottom of a 13x9-inch glass baking pan.
Lay out 4 noodles over the sauce and top with 1 C. of the cheese mixture, followed by 1 C. of sauce and 2/3 C. of mozzarella cheese.
Repeat the layers twice.
With a piece of heavy-duty foil, cover the baking pan and bake for around 30 minutes.
Uncover the baking pan and bake for around 15 minutes.
Take it out of the oven and set it aside for around 10 minutes before enjoying it.

INGREDIENTS REQUIRED:

- Bulk Italian pork sausage – 1 lb. (455 g)
- Medium-sized onion – 1, cut up
- Garlic clove – 1, crushed
- Diced tomatoes – 1 (14-oz.) (390-g) can (with juices)
- Tomato sauce – 1 (15-oz.) (425-g) can
- Fresh parsley – 4 tbsp., cut up and divided
- White sugar – 1 tsp.
- Lasagna noodles – 12
- Ricotta cheese – 1 (15-oz.) (425-g) container
- Parmesan cheese – ½ C. (55 g), grated and divided
- Fresh oregano leaves – 2 tbsp., cut up
- Mozzarella cheese – 2 C. (230 g), shredded

NOTES

BEANS & GRAINS RECIPES

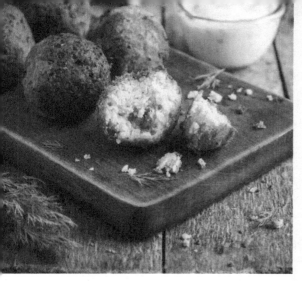

Falafel with Tzatziki

Prep period: 20 mins.
Cook period: 12 mins.
Serves: 8

Per Serving: Calories 280, Fat 19.2
Carbs 18.5g, Protein 10.7g

INGREDIENTS REQUIRED:

For the Falafel:
- Dried chickpeas – 1 lb. (455 g)
- Small-sized onion – 1, roughly cut up
- Fresh parsley – ¼ C., cut up
- Garlic cloves – 4, peeled
- Chickpea flour – 1½ tbsp.
- Salt – as desired
- Cayenne pepper powder – ½ tsp.
- Olive oil – ½ C. (120 ml)

For the Tzatziki Sauce:
- Large-sized cucumber – 1, peel removed and grated
- Salt – as desired
- Plain Greek yogurt – 2 C. (500 g)
- Lemon juice – 1 tbsp. freshly squeezed
- Garlic cloves – 4, minced
- Fresh dill – 2 tbsp. cut up
- Fresh mint leaves – 1 tbsp. cut up
- Cayenne pepper powder – 1 pinch of
- Ground black pepper – as desired

PROCEDURE:

1. For the falafel: soak the chickpeas int large-sized basin of water overnight.
2. Then, drain the chickpeas and rinse thoroughly.
3. Put the chickpeas and remnant ingredients into an electric food processor and process them thorougl
4. Place the falafel mixture into a basin.
5. With plastic wrap, cover the basin of mixture and put it into your fridge fo around 1-2 hours.
6. In the meantime, for the tzatziki: lay a colander in the sink.
7. Place the cucumber into the colander and sprinkle with salt.
8. Let it drain for around 10-15 minutes
9. With your hands, squeeze the cucum thoroughly.
10. Put the cucumber and remnant ingredients into a large-sized basin a blend to incorporate.
11. Cover the basin of tzatziki and put it your fridge to chill for at least 1 hour
12. Shape the chickpea mixture into sma sized balls.
13. Sizzle oil into a large-sized wok to 37 (190 ºC).
14. Cook the falafels in 2 batches for aro 5-6 minutes.
15. With a slotted spoon, shift the falafel onto a paper towel-lined plate to dra
16. Enjoy the falafels alongside tzatziki.

Chickpeas & Veggie Tagine

Prep period: 15 mins.

Cook period: 1 hr.

Serves: 6

er Serving: Calories 492, Fat 14.2g, Carbs 74.6g, Protein 20.2g

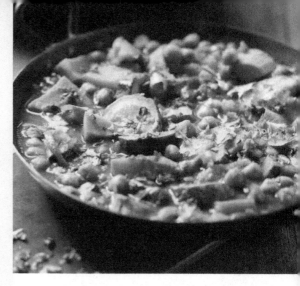

PROCEDURE:

Sizzle oil into a large, heavy-bottomed Dutch oven on the burner at medium-high heat.
Cook the onions for around 4-6 minutes.
Put in garlic and cook for around 1 minute.
Put in the potatoes, zucchini, spices, and salt and blend.
Cook for around 5-7 minutes, stirring frequently.
Put in the tomatoes, apricot, and broth and stir.
Cook for around 10 minutes.
Turn the heat to low.
Cook with the cover for another 20-25 minutes.
Put in chickpeas and stir.
Cook for around 5 minutes.
Blend in lemon juice and parsley, and enjoy right away.

INGREDIENTS REQUIRED:

- Olive oil – ¼ C. (60 ml)
- Medium-sized onions – 2, cut up
- Garlic cloves – 8-10, cut up
- Large-sized sweet potato – 1, peel removed and cubed
- Large-sized russet potatoes – 2, peel removed and cubed
- Medium-sized zucchinis – 2, cut up
- Harissa spice blend – 1 tbsp.
- Ground coriander – 1 tsp.
- Ground cinnamon – 1 tsp.
- Ground turmeric – ½ tsp.
- Salt – as desired
- Whole peeled tomatoes – 1 (15-oz.) (425-g) can
- Dried apricots – ½ C. (85 g), cut up
- Vegetable broth – 4 C. (960 ml)
- Chickpeas – 1 (14-oz.) (400-g) can, liquid removed
- Lemon juice – 2 tbsp. (30 ml), freshly squeezed
- Fresh parsley – ¼ C. (5 g), cut up

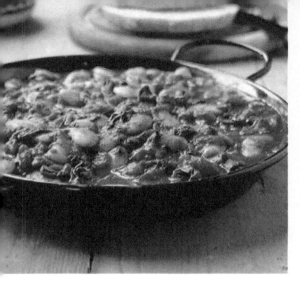

Beans, Tomato & Spinach Bake

Prep period: 15 mins.
Cook period: 1 hr. 55 mins.
Serves: 4

Per Serving: Calories 180, Fat 7.5g,
Carbs 32.7g, Protein 8.9g

INGREDIENTS REQUIRED:

- Dried lima beans – 1 C. (180 g)
- Bay leaf – 1
- Vegetable bouillon cube – 1
- Olive oil – 3 tbsp. (45 ml)
- Small-sized onion – 1, finely cut up
- Garlic cloves – 3, minced
- Diced tomatoes – 1 (15-oz.) (425-g) can
- Tomato paste – ¼ C. (75 g)
- Maple syrup – 1 tbsp.
- Red wine vinegar – 1 tsp.
- Dried oregano – 1 tsp.
- Dried thyme – 1 tsp.
- Ground nutmeg – 1 pinch
- Salt and ground black pepper – as desired
- Fresh spinach – 2 C. (60 g), cut up

PROCEDURE:

1. Soak the beans in a large basin water for around 8 hours.
2. Then, drain the beans and rinse thoroughly.
3. Put the beans and bay leaf into large pot of water on the burner at high heat.
4. Cook the mixture until boiling.
5. Turn the heat to around medium.
6. Cook for around 30 minutes.
7. Drain the beans, reserving 1 C. of cooking liquid.
8. Dissolve the bouillon cube in the reserved hot cooking liquid.
9. For preheating: set your oven a 375 °F (190 °C).
10. Sizzle oil into a large-sized Dutch oven on the burner at medium heat.
11. Cook the onion and garlic for 6-8 minutes.

....

....

....

....

....

PROCEDURE:

....

12. Blend in the bouillon cube mixture, tomatoes, tomato paste, maple syrup, vinegar, dried herbs, nutmeg, salt, and pepper, and turn the heat to medium-high.

....

....

13. Cook the mixture until boiling.

....

14. Turn the heat to around low.

15. Cook for around 10-12 minutes.

....

16. Stir in beans and take off the burner.

....

17. With a piece of heavy-duty foil, cover the pot and shift into the oven.

....

18. Bake for around 30-40 minutes.

19. Take off the foil from the Dutch oven and bake for around 10-15 minutes

....

20. Take off the pot of beans mixture from the oven and immediately stir in spinach.

....

21. Cover the pot for around 10 minutes before enjoying.

....

....

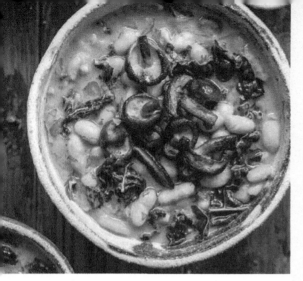

Creamy Beans with Veggies

Prep period: 10 mins.
Cook period: 4 mins.
Serves: 4

Per Serving: Calories 313, Fat 8.1g,
Carbs 45.7g, Protein 16.9g

INGREDIENTS REQUIRED:

- Olive oil – 2 tbsp. (30 ml)
- Large-sized onion – 1, cut up
- Fresh mushrooms – 8 oz. (220 g), sliced
- White beans – 2 (14-oz.) (400-g) cans
- Vegetable broth – 2 C. (480 ml)
- Fresh spinach – 2 C. (60 g), cut up
- Heavy cream – 1 C. (240 g)
- Salt and ground black pepper – as desired

PROCEDURE:

1. Sizzle oil into a large-sized pot on a burner at around medium heat.
2. Cook the onion for around 4-5 minutes.
3. Put in mushrooms and blend.
4. Cook for around 5 minutes.
5. Put in beans and broth and stir
6. Cook the mixture until boiling
7. Turn the heat to low.
8. Cook for around 10 minutes.
9. Put in spinach and cream and stir.
10. Cook for around 3-5 minutes.
11. Stir in salt and pepper and take off the burner.
12. Enjoy right away.

Lentil & Quinoa Stew

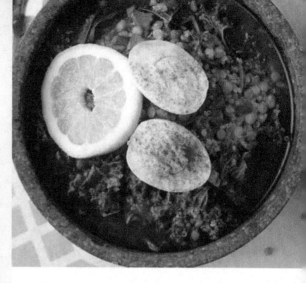

Prep period: 15 mins.
Cook period: 35 mins.
Serves: 6

Per Serving: Calories 283, Fat 5.1g,
Carbs 43.3g, Protein 17.1g

PROCEDURE:

Sizzle oil into a large-sized pot on a burner at medium heat.
Cook the celery, onion, and carrot for around 4-5 minutes.
Put in garlic and cook for around 1 minute.
Put in remnant ingredients except for the spinach and stir.
Cook the mixture until boiling.
Turn the heat to low.
Cook with the cover for 20 minutes.
Put in spinach and stir.
Cook for 3-4 minutes.
Stir in salt and pepper and take off the burner.
Enjoy right away.

INGREDIENTS REQUIRED:

- Olive oil – 1 tbsp. (15 ml)
- Medium-sized carrots – 3, peel removed and cut up
- Celery stalks – 3, cut up
- Medium-sized onion – 1, cut up
- Garlic cloves – 4, minced
- Tomatoes – 4 C. (800 g), cut up
- Red lentils – 1 C. (210 g), rinsed
- Quinoa – ½ C. (95 g), rinsed
- Ground cumin – 1 tsp.
- Red chili powder – 1 tsp.
- Vegetable broth – 5 C. (1200 ml)
- Fresh kale – 3 C. (165 g), tough ribs removed and cut up
- Salt and ground black pepper – as desired

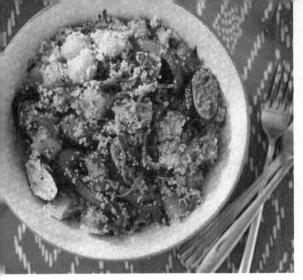

Couscous & Veggie Pilaf

Prep period: 15 mins.
Cook period: 22 mins.
Serves: 4

Per Serving: Calories 493, Fat 18g,
Carbs 68.8g, Protein 16g

INGREDIENTS REQUIRED:

- Olive oil – 3 tbsp. (15 ml)
- Medium-sized onion – 1, cut up
- Medium-sized parsnip – 1, peel removed and thinly slivered
- Medium-sized carrot – 1, peel removed and thinly slivered
- Medium-sized zucchini – 1, cut into ¾-inch pieces
- Medium-sized bell peppers – 2, cut into ¾-inch pieces
- Garlic cloves – 2, minced
- Ground cumin – 1 tsp.
- Red pepper flakes – 1 tsp.
- Couscous – 1½ C. (250 g)
- Salt and ground black pepper – as needed
- Dried apricots – ½ C. (80 g), cut up
- Vegetable broth – 2¼ C. (500 ml)
- Fresh parsley – ¼ C. (5 g) cut up

PROCEDURE:

1. Sizzle oil into a large-sized cast-iron wok on the burner at medium-high heat.
2. Cook the onion for 4-5 minute
3. Put in parsnip and carrot and blend.
4. Cook for around 4-5 minutes.
5. Put in zucchini, bell peppers, garlic, and spices and blend.
6. Cook for 4-5 minutes.
7. Put in the couscous and blend
8. Cook for around 1½-2 minute stirring from time to time.
9. Put in apricots and broth and stir.
10. Cook with the cover for aroun 5 minutes.
11. Take off the pot of pilaf from t burner and fluff the couscous thoroughly with a fork.
12. Blend in parsley and enjoy.

Barley & Mushroom Risotto

Prep period: 15 mins.
Cook period: 1 hr. 5 mins.
Serves: 4

Per Serving: Calories 187, Fat 7.9g,
Carbs 26g, Protein 5g

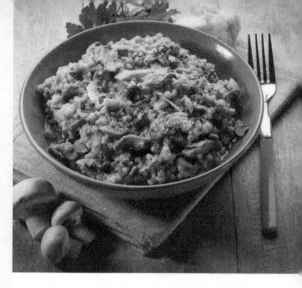

PROCEDURE:

Put the barley and broth into a pot on a burner at medium-high heat.
Cook the mixture until boiling.
Turn the heat to low.
Cook with the cover on for around 45 minutes.
Sizzle 1 tbsp. of oil into a large-sized wok on a burner at high heat.
Cook the garlic for 1 minute.
Put in cooked barley and stir.
Cook for around 3 minutes.
Take off the wok of barley mixture from the burner and set it aside.
Sizzle remnant oil into another wok on the burner at medium heat.
Cook the onion for around 4-5 minutes.
Put in mushrooms and stir.
Stir-fry for 5-6 minutes.
Put in remnant ingredients and stir.
Cook for around 2 minutes.
Put in barley mixture and stir.
Cook for 2-3 minutes.
Enjoy right away.

INGREDIENTS REQUIRED:

- Pearl barley – ½ C. (100 g)
- Vegetable broth – 1¼ C. (300 ml)
- Olive oil – 2 tbsp. (30 ml), divided
- Garlic cloves – 2, minced
- Onions – ½ C. (60 g), cut up
- Fresh mushrooms – 1½ C. (190 g), sliced
- Fresh parsley – 2 tbsp., cut up
- Fresh mint leaves – 2 tbsp., cut up
- White sugar – 1 tsp.
- Soy sauce – 1 tbsp. (15 ml)

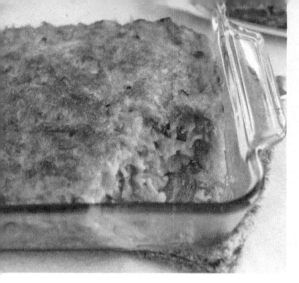

Rice & Lentil Gratin

Prep period: 15 mins.
Cook period: 1 hr. 10 mins.
Serves: 6

Per Serving: Calories 261, Fat 6.4g,
Carbs 32.1g, Protein 12.8g

INGREDIENTS REQUIRED:

- Unsalted butter – 2 tbsp. (30 g)
- Leeks – 3, halved and cut up
- Dry white wine – ½ C. (120 ml)
- Chicken broth – 1 C. (240 ml)
- Salt and ground black pepper – as desired
- Heavy cream – ¼ C. (60 g)
- Olive oil baking spray
- Canned lentils – 1 C. (200 g), liquid removed and rinsed
- Cooked long-grain white rice – ¾ C. (130 g)
- Panko breadcrumbs – ¼ C. (40 g)
- Parmesan cheese – ¼ C. (30 g), grated

PROCEDURE:

1. Sizzle butter into a wok on the burner at medium heat.
2. Cook the leeks for around 5-6 minutes.
3. Put in wine and stir.
4. Cook for around 2-3 minutes.
5. Stir in broth, salt, and pepper, and immediately cover the wok.
6. Cook for 25-30 minutes.
7. For preheating: set your oven a 400 °F (205 °C).
8. Spray a casserole dish with baking spray.
9. Put the cream into the wok of leek mixture and blend thoroughly.
10. Cook for 3-5 minutes, stirring the time.
11. Take off from the burner and blend in lentils and rice.
12. Place the mixture into the casserole dish and sprinkle with breadcrumbs, followed by cheese.
13. Bake for around 15 minutes.
14. Take it off the oven and set it aside for around 5 minutes before enjoying it.

Green Peas Risotto

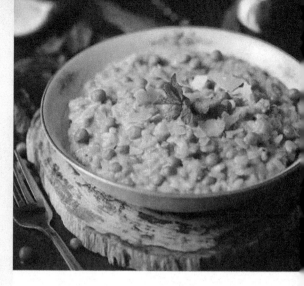

Prep period: 15 mins.
Cook period: 35 mins.
Serves: 2

er Serving: Calories 587, Fat 23.9g,
Carbs 65.3g, Protein 17.4g

PROCEDURE:

Sizzle oil into a pot on a burner at medium heat.
Cook the onion and leek for around 5 minutes.
Put in rice and blend.
Cook for 2 minutes.
Put in wine and stir.
Cook for 2-3 minutes.
Put in ½ C. of broth and blend.
Cook until all the broth is absorbed, stirring from time to time.
Repeat this process by adding ¾ C. of broth at one time, stirring from time to time or until all the broth is absorbed. (This procedure will take about 20 minutes).
Take it off the burner and stir in remnant ingredients to incorporate them thoroughly.
Return the pot to the burner at medium-high heat.
Cook for 5 minutes.
Enjoy right away.

INGREDIENTS REQUIRED:

- Olive oil – 1 tbsp. (15 ml)
- Small-sized onion – 1, sliced
- Leek – ½, sliced
- Risotto rice – ½ C. (110 g), rinsed and liquid removed
- White wine – ½ C. (120 ml)
- Vegetable broth – 2-3 C. (480-720 ml)
- Frozen green peas – 1 C. (160 g)
- Cream cheese – 2½ oz. (70 g)
- Heavy cream – 1/3 C. (90 g)
- Soy sauce – 2 tbsp. (30 ml)
- Worcestershire sauce – 2 tbsp. (30 ml)
- Fresh parsley – 2 tbsp., cut up

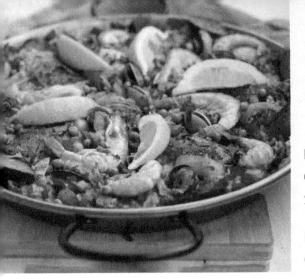

Rice & Seafood Paella

Prep period: 20 mins.
Cook period: 1 hr.
Serves: 4

Per Serving: Calories 456, Fat 6.8g
Carbs 76.7g, Protein 21.1g

INGREDIENTS REQUIRED:

- Olive oil – 1 tbsp. (15 ml)
- Medium-sized bell pepper – 1, seeded and finely cut up
- Large-sized onion – 1, finely cut up
- Garlic cloves – 4, minced
- Short-grain white rice – 1½ C. (300 g)
- Ground turmeric – ½ tsp.
- Paprika – 1 tsp.
- Diced tomatoes – 1 (14-oz.) (400 g) can
- Saffron threads – 2 pinches, crushed
- Chicken broth – 3 C. (720 ml)
- Mussels – 12, cleaned
- Shrimp – 12, peeled and deveined
- Frozen green peas – ½ C. (80 g), thawed
- Fresh parsley – ¼ C. (5 g), cut up
- Lemon – 1, cut into wedges

PROCEDURE:

1. Sizzle oil into a deep pan on a burner at medium-high heat.
2. Cook the bell pepper, onion, ar garlic for around 3 minutes.
3. Put in rice, turmeric, and paprika and stir.
4. Cook for 1-2 minutes.
5. Put in tomatoes, saffron, and broth and stir.
6. Cook the mixture until boiling
7. Turn the heat to around low.
8. Cook with the cover on for around 20 minutes.
9. Lay out the mussels, shrimp, a peas on top of the rice mixture
10. Cook with the cover on for around 10-15 minutes.
11. Enjoy right away with the garnishing of parsley and lemc wedges.

POULTRY RECIPES

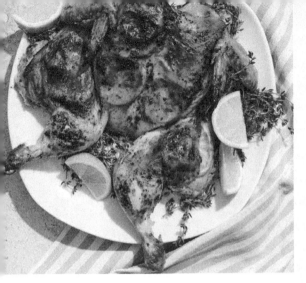

Herbed Whole Chicken

Prep period: 15 mins.
Cook period: 50 mins.
Serves: 6

Per Serving: Calories 644, Fat 29.6
Carbs 1.6g, Protein 87.8g

INGREDIENTS REQUIRED:

- Whole chicken – 1 (4-lb.) (1 kg 820 g), neck and giblets removed
- Fresh ginger – 2 tsp., finely cut up
- Garlic cloves – 4, cut up
- Fresh thyme bunch – 1
- Fresh rosemary bunch – 1
- Paprika – ½ tsp.
- Ground cumin – ½ tsp.
- Salt and ground black pepper – as desired
- Lemon juice – ¼ C. (60 ml), freshly squeezed
- Olive oil – 3 tbsp. (45 ml)

PROCEDURE:

1. Lay out the chicken onto a large-sized chopping board, breast-side down.
2. With a kitchen shear, start from the thigh, cut along one side of the backbone, and turn the chicken around.
3. Now, cut along the other side and discard the backbone.
4. Change the side and open it like a book.
5. Pound the backbone firmly to flat
6. Put remnant ingredients except for chicken into an electric food processor and process to form a smooth mixture.
7. Put the marinade mixture into a large baking pan.
8. Put in chicken and coat with marinade generously.
9. With plastic wrap, cover the bakir pan and put it into your fridge to marinate overnight.
10. For preheating: set your oven at 4 °F (230 °C).
11. Lay out a rack into a roasting pan
12. Take out the chicken from the fri and discard the excess marinade.
13. Lay out the chicken on the rack o the roasting pan, skin side down.
14. Roast for around 25 minutes.
15. Flip the chicken and roast for aro 25 minutes.
16. Take the roasting pan of chicken out of the oven and place it onto ; platter for around 10 minutes bef carving.
17. Cut the chicken into serving port and enjoy.

Lemony Chicken Drumsticks

Prep period: 10 mins.

Cook period: 40 mins.

Serves: 6

er Serving: Calories 340, Fat 14.6g, Carbs 2.5g, Protein 47.2g

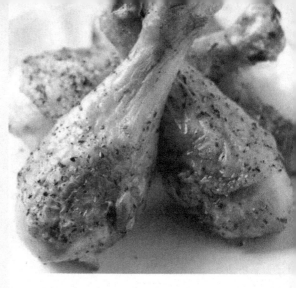

PROCEDURE:

Rub the chicken drumsticks with salt generously.

Lay the chicken drumsticks onto a baking tray and put into your fridge for 3-4 hours.

Put the chicken drumsticks, oil, lemon juice, onion, garlic, lemon zest, oregano, spices, and pepper into a large-sized zip-lock bag. Seal the bag and shake to coat thoroughly.

Put into your fridge to marinate for around 30 minutes.

For preheating: set your oven at 450 °F (230 °C).

Lightly spray a baking pan with a baking spray.

Place the chicken drumsticks with marinade into the baking pan.

Arrange lemon slices between the drumsticks.

Bake for 35 minutes.

Now set your oven to broiler.

Broil for around 3-5 minutes.

Enjoy right away.

INGREDIENTS REQUIRED:

- Chicken drumsticks – 6
- Salt – as desired
- Olive oil – 2 tbsp. (30 ml)
- Lemon juice – 2 tbsp. (30 ml), freshly squeezed
- Medium-sized onion – ½, cut into wedges
- Garlic cloves – 6, cut up
- Lemon zest – 2 tsp., grated
- Dried oregano – 1 tsp.
- Ground coriander – 1 tsp.
- Ground cumin – ½ tsp.
- Sweet paprika – ½ tsp.
- Ground black pepper – as desired
- Olive oil baking spray
- Lemon – 1, sliced

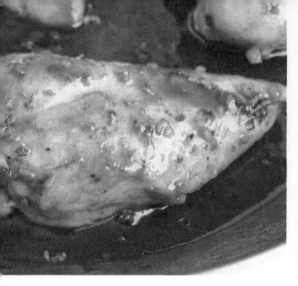

Glazed Chicken Breasts

Prep period: 10 mins.
Cook period: 33 mins.
Serves: 4

Per Serving: Calories 465, Fat 15.1g
Carbs 44.4g, Protein 39g

INGREDIENTS REQUIRED:

- Fresh parsley – 2 tbsp., cut up
- Garlic cloves – 5, minced
- Brown sugar – ½ C. (85 g)
- Apricot jam – ½ C. (160 g)
- White wine – ½ C. (120 ml)
- Red wine vinegar – 1/3 C. (90 ml)
- Caper brine – 1 tbsp. (15 ml)
- Olive oil – 2 tbsp. (30 ml)
- Boneless & skinless chicken breasts – 4 (6-oz.) (150-g)
- Fresh parsley – 2 tbsp. (2½ g) cut up

PROCEDURE:

1. For preheating: set your oven at 350 °F (175 °C).
2. Put the parsley and remnant ingredients except for oil and chicken breasts into a large basin and blend to incorporate thoroughly. Set it aside.
3. Sizzle oil into a large wok on the burner at around medium-high heat.
4. Sear the chicken breasts for around 1½ minutes per side.
5. Take off the burner and place the chicken in a baking pan.
6. Place the jam mixture on top.
7. Bake for around 20-30 minutes
8. Enjoy right away with the garnishing of parsley.

Chicken Parmigiana

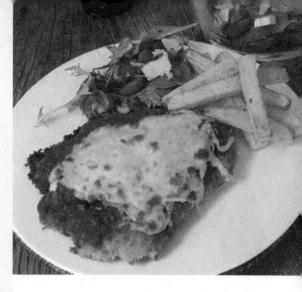

Prep period: 15 mins.

Cook period: 26 mins.

Serves: 4

Per Serving: Calories 458, Fat 25.4g, Carbs: 7.9g, Protein 50.4g

PROCEDURE:

For preheating: set your oven at 375 °F (190 °C)

Lay out 1 chicken breast between 2 pieces of parchment paper.

With a meat mallet, pound the chicken breast into ½-inch thickness

Repeat with the remnant chicken breasts.

Put the whisked egg into a shallow dish.

Put the almond flour, Parmesan, parsley, spices, salt, and pepper into another shallow dish and blend to incorporate.

Dip each chicken breast into the whisked egg and then coat it with the flour mixture.

Sizzle oil into a deep wok on the burner at around medium-high heat.

Cook the chicken breasts for around 3 minutes per side.

With a slotted spoon, shift the chicken breasts onto a paper towel-lined plate.

Put about ½ C. of tomato sauce in the bottom of a casserole dish and spread evenly.

Lay out the chicken breasts over tomato sauce.

Top with the remnant tomato sauce, followed by mozzarella cheese.

Bake for around 20 minutes.

Take it out of the oven and enjoy it right away with the garnishing of parsley.

INGREDIENTS REQUIRED:

- Boneless & skinless chicken breasts – 5 (6-oz.) (150-g)
- Large-sized egg – 1, whisked
- Superfine blanched almond flour – ½ C. (50 g)
- Parmesan cheese – ¼ C. (30 g), grated
- Dried parsley – ½ tsp.
- Paprika – ½ tsp.
- Garlic powder – ½ tsp.
- Salt and ground black pepper – as desired
- Olive oil – ¼ C. (60 ml)
- Tomato sauce – 1 C. (300 g)
- Mozzarella cheese – 5 oz. (140 g), thinly sliced
- Fresh parsley – 2 tbsp. cut up

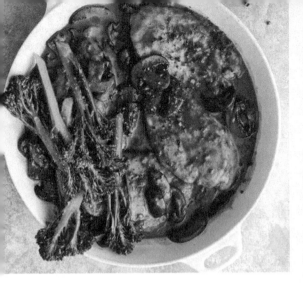

Chicken Marsala

Prep period: 15 mins.

Cook period: 30 mins.

Serves: 4

Per Serving: Calories 547, Fat 32.7
Carbs 17.6g, Protein 37.8g

INGREDIENTS REQUIRED:

- All-purpose flour – ½ C. (65 g)
- Garlic cloves – 3 powder
- Salt and ground black pepper – as desired
- Boneless & skinless chicken breasts – 4 (4-oz.) (110-g), pounded slightly
- Olive oil – 2 tbsp. (30 ml)
- Unsalted butter – 3 tbsp. (42 g), divided
- Fresh Cremini mushrooms – 8 oz. (220 g), sliced
- Garlic cloves – 4, minced
- Dry Marsala wine – ¾ C. (180 ml)
- Chicken broth – 1¼ C. (300 ml)
- Heavy cream – ¾ C. (180 g)
- Fresh parsley – 2 tbsp., cut up

PROCEDURE:

1. Put the flour, garlic powder, sal and pepper into a shallow basiı and blend thoroughly.
2. Coat the chicken breasts with flour mixture and then shake o excess.
3. Sizzle 2 tbsp. of butter and oil into a wok on the burner at medium-high heat.
4. Cook the chicken breasts in 2 batches for around 3-4 minute per side.
5. With a slotted spoon, shift the chicken breasts onto a warm plate and cover with a piece of heavy-duty foil to keep warm.
6. Sizzle the remnant butter in the same wok on the burner at around medium heat.
7. Cook the mushrooms for 2-3 minutes, stirring frequently.
8. Put in garlic and cook for around 1 minute, stirring all tl time.
9. Put in Marsala and the broth a stir.
10. Cook for around 10-15 minut
11. Put in chicken and cream and stir.
12. Cook for around 3 minutes.
13. Enjoy right away with the garnishing of parsley.

Chicken Margarita

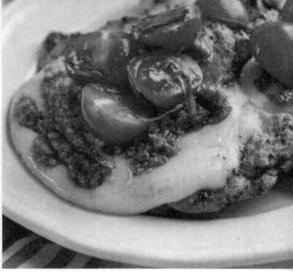

Prep period: 15 mins.
Cook period: 26 mins.
Serves: 4

Per Serving: Calories 913, Fat 57.7g,
Carbs: 6.6g, Protein 89.9g

PROCEDURE:

For preheating: set your oven at 350 °F (175 °C).
Put the chicken breasts and marinade into a resealable bag. Seal the bag and shake to coat thoroughly.
Put into your fridge to marinate for at least 30 minutes.
Sizzle oil into a large cast-iron wok on the burner at medium-high heat.
Cook the chicken breasts for 7-8 minutes per side.
In the meantime, cook the butter, lemon juice, and garlic in a small pot for 2 minutes, stirring all the time.
With a slotted spoon, shift the chicken breasts into a baking pan and brush each with butter mixture.
Place 2 mozzarella slices over each chicken breast, followed by 1 tbsp. of pesto.
Bake for 7-10 minutes.
Take out of the oven and place the chicken breasts onto serving plates.
Brush with any remnant butter mixture and garnish with basil. Enjoy alongside tomatoes.

INGREDIENTS REQUIRED:

- Boneless & skinless chicken breasts – 4 (8-oz.) (220-g), pounded slightly
- Chicken marinade – 1 C. (300 g)
- Olive oil – 2 tbsp. (30 ml)
- Unsalted butter – 1/3 C. (85 g), cut into pieces
- Lemon juice – 4 tsp. (20 ml) freshly squeezed
- Garlic cloves – 4, minced
- Mozzarella cheese slices – 8
- Pesto – ½ C. (70 g)
- Grape tomatoes – 1 C. (150 g), halved
- Fresh basil – ¼ C. (5 g), thinly sliced

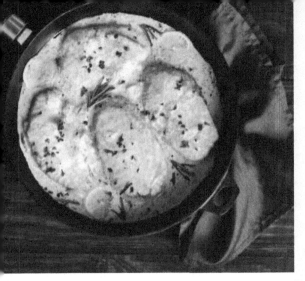

Chicken in Creamy Sauce

Prep period: 15 mins.
Cook period: 25 mins.
Serves: 4

Per Serving: Calories 592, Fat 34.2
Carbs 7.7g, Protein 60.7g

INGREDIENTS REQUIRED:

- Boneless & skinless chicken breasts, – 4 (7-oz.) (200 g), pounded
- Salt and ground black pepper – as desired
- Olive oil – 1 tbsp. (15 ml)
- Unsalted butter – 3 tbsp. (40 g)
- Small-sized shallot – 1, finely cut up
- Garlic cloves – 4, minced
- All-purpose flour – 2 tbsp. (15 g)
- Half-and-half – 1 C. (240 g)
- Chicken broth – ½ C. (120 ml)
- Lemon juice – 3 tbsp. (45 ml), freshly squeezed
- Fresh parsley – 2 tbsp., cut up
- Small-sized lemon – 1, thinly sliced

PROCEDURE:

1. Rub each chicken breast with s and pepper generously.
2. Sizzle oil into a large-sized wok on the burner at around medium-high heat.
3. Cook the chicken breasts for around 6-7 minutes per side.
4. With a slotted spoon, shift the chicken breasts onto a plate.
5. Sizzle butter in the same wok the burner at medium heat.
6. Cook the shallot, garlic, salt, a pepper for 1 minute, stirring from time to time.
7. Put in the flour and stir.
8. Cook for around 1 minute, stirring all the time.
9. Put in half-and-half and broth and stir.
10. Cook the mixture until boiling
11. Stir in cooked chicken breasts and turn the heat at around lo
12. Cook for 3-4 minutes.
13. Stir in lemon juice and take of the burner.
14. Enjoy right away with the garnishing of parsley and lem slices.

Baked Chicken with Olives

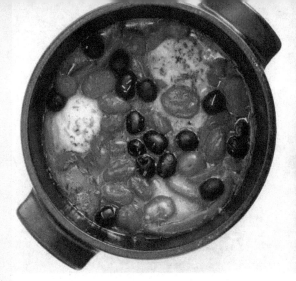

Prep period: 10 mins.
Cook period: 21 mins.
Serves: 4

er Serving: Calories 341, Fat 18.2g,
Carbs: 5.7g, Protein 37.5g

PROCEDURE:

For preheating: set your oven at 375 °F (190 °C)

Into a basin, put the dried herbs, salt and pepper and blend thoroughly.

Rub the chicken breasts with the herb mixture

Sizzle oil into a cast-iron wok on the burner at around medium-high heat.

Cook the chicken for around 3 minutes per side.

With a slotted spoon, shift the chicken breasts onto a plate.

Put the garlic, broth, and lemon juice in the same wok on the burner at medium heat.

Cook for 5 minutes.

Take it off the burner and stir in cooked chicken breasts.

Spread the olives, tomatoes, and onions on top of the chicken mixture.

Bake for around 10 minutes.

Take it out of the oven and set it aside for around 5-10 minutes.

Enjoy with the topping of feta cheese.

INGREDIENTS REQUIRED:

- Dried basil – 1 tsp.
- Dried parsley – ½ tsp.
- Salt and ground black pepper – as desired
- Chicken breasts – 2 (8-oz.) (225-g), cut in half lengthwise
- Olive oil – 1 tbsp. (15 ml)
- Garlic cloves – 2, minced
- Chicken broth – 1 C. (240 ml)
- Lemon juice – 1 tbsp. (15 ml), freshly squeezed
- Cherry tomatoes – 1 C. (150 g), quartered
- Black olives – ½ C. (90 g), finely cut up
- Onions – ½ C. (60 g), finely cut up
- Feta cheese – ½ C. (55 g), crumbled

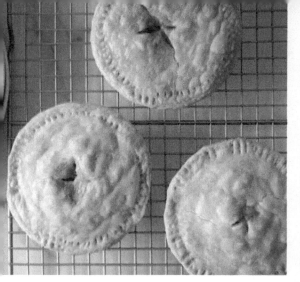

Turkey Pot Pies

Prep period: 20 mins.
Cook period: 35 mins.
Serves: 6

Per Serving: Calories 480, Fat 23.7g
Carbs 42.5g, Protein 25.7g

INGREDIENTS REQUIRED:

For the Filling:
- Olive oil – 2 tsp. (10 ml)
- Medium-sized onions – 2, thinly sliced
- Garlic cloves – 3, minced
- All-purpose flour – 3 tbsp. (25 g)
- Chicken broth – 1¼ C. (300 ml)
- Diced tomatoes – 1 (14-oz.) (400-g) can (with juices)
- Cooked turkey breast – 2½ C. (400 g), cubed
- Water-packed artichoke hearts – 1 (14-oz.) (400-g) can, rinsed, liquid removed, and sliced
- Ripe olives – ½ C. (90 g), pitted and halved
- Pepperoncini – ¼ C. (30 g), sliced
- Dried oregano – 1 tsp.
- Ground black pepper – as desired

For the Crust:
- Frozen pizza dough loaf – 12 oz. (340 g), thawed
- Large-sized egg white – 1
- Dried oregano – ¼ tsp.

PROCEDURE:

1. Soak the beans in a large basin For preheating: set your oven at 425 °F (220 °C).
2. For the filling: sizzle oil into a Dutch oven on the burner at medium heat.
3. Cook the onions for 4-5 minute
4. Stir in garlic and cook for 2 minutes.
5. In the meantime, put the flour and broth into a small basin an stir to dissolve thoroughly.
6. Slowly put the flour mixture in the wok, stirring all the time.
7. Put in tomatoes and stir.
8. Cook the mixture until boiling
9. Cook for around 2 minutes, stirring all the time.
10. Take off from the burner and stir in turkey, artichokes, olives pepperoncini, oregano, and pepper.
11. Divide turkey mixture into 6 ramekins.
12. For the crust: put the egg white and oregano into a small-sized basin and whisk slightly.

PROCEDURE:

3. Roll the dough and place about 2 oz. (56 g) on top of the filling in each ramekin.
4. Press the edges of each dough to seal the filling.
5. With a knife, cut slits in each dough.
6. Brush the top of the dough with the egg-white mixture.
. Lay out the ramekins onto a baking tray.
. Bake for around 18-22 minutes.
. Remove the ramekins from the oven and set them aside for around 5 minutes before enjoying.

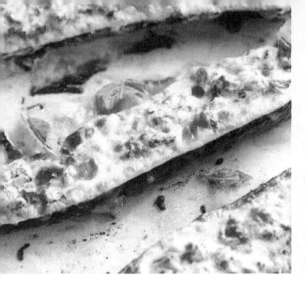

Turkey Stuffed Zucchini

Prep period: 15 mins.
Cook period: 20 mins.
Serves: 8

Per Serving: Calories 218, Fat 13.9g
Carbs 8.5g, Protein 19.2g

INGREDIENTS REQUIRED:

- Large-sized zucchinis – 4, halved lengthwise
- Olive oil – 3 tbsp. (45 ml), divided
- Ground turkey – 1 lb. (455 g)
- Medium-sized onion – 1, grated
- Garlic cloves – 3, minced
- Dried oregano – 2 tsp.
- Lemon pepper seasoning – 1 tbsp.
- Salt – as desired
- Sun-dried tomatoes – ¼ C. (30 g), cut up
- Feta cheese – ½ C. (55 g), crumbled

PROCEDURE:

1. For preheating: set your oven at 3 °F (175 °C).
2. With a spoon, scoop out the insic of the zucchini to create a boat.
3. Lay out the zucchini halves onto baking tray and cut side up.
4. Drizzle the halves with 2 tbsp. of oil and then sprinkle with salt an pepper.
5. Bake for around 10 minutes.
6. In the meantime, sizzle remnant oil into a large-sized wok on the burner at around medium-high heat.
7. Cook the turkey for around 6-7 minutes, stirring from time to ti
8. Put in onion, garlic, oregano, len pepper, and salt, and blend.
9. Cook for 2-3 minutes.
10. Take off from the burner and set aside.
11. Take the baking tray out of the o and stuff each zucchini half with the turkey mixture.
12. Sprinkle each boat with feta che followed by sun-dried tomatoes.
13. Bake for around 5-10 minutes.
14. Enjoy right away.

MEAT RECIPES

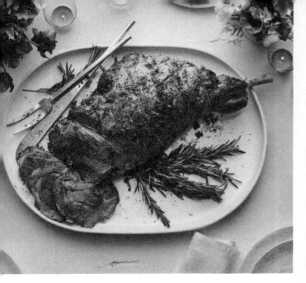

Rosemary Leg of Lamb

Prep period: 15 mins.
Cook period: 1½ hrs.
Serves: 8

Per Serving: Calories 610, Fat 29.6
Carbs 2g, Protein 80.1g

INGREDIENTS REQUIRED:

- Fresh rosemary – ¼ C. (5 g), minced
- Garlic cloves – 4, minced
- Lemon zest – 1 tsp., finely grated
- Ground coriander – 2 tsp.
- Ground cumin – 2 tsp.
- Paprika – 2 tsp.
- Red pepper flakes – 2 tsp., finely crushed
- Ground allspice – ½ tsp.
- Olive oil – 1/3 C. (90 ml)
- Bone-in leg of lamb – 1 (5-lb.) (2 kg 275 g), trimmed
- Olive oil baking spray

PROCEDURE:

1. Put the rosemary and remnan ingredients except the leg of lamb into a large basin and sti thoroughly.
2. Coat the leg of lamb with the marinade mixture generously.
3. With a plastic wrap, cover the leg of lamb and put it into you fridge to marinate for around 6-8 hours.
4. Take out of the fridge and kee at room temperature for arou 30 minutes before roasting.
5. For preheating: lay out a rack the center of the oven.
6. Set your oven at 350 °F (175 °
7. Lay out a rack in the roasting pan and then spray it lightly ʋ baking spray.
8. Place the leg of lamb over the rack in the roasting pan.
9. Roast for around 1¼-1½ hou rotating the pan once halfway through.
10. Take out of the oven and plac the leg of lamb onto a choppi board for around 10-15 minu
11. Cut the leg of lamb into servi portions and enjoy.

Braised Lamb Shanks

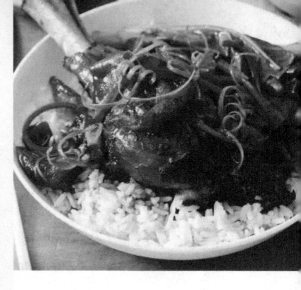

Prep period: 10 mins.
Cook period: 2 hrs. 40 mins.
Serves: 2

Per Serving: Calories 811, Fat 53g,
Carbs 5.4g, Protein 74.3g

PROCEDURE:

For preheating: set your oven at 325 ºF (165 ºC).
Sizzle oil into an ovenproof pot on a burner at medium-high heat.
Cook the lamb shanks for around 3-4 minutes, flipping once halfway through.
With a slotted spoon, shift the shanks onto a plate.
Cook the onion, garlic, spices, and salt in the same pot for around 40-60 seconds.
Put in wine and turn the heat to high.
Cook for around 1-2 minutes, scraping up the brown bits
Put in cooked shanks, broth, and bay leaves and blend.
Cook the mixture until boiling.
Immediately cover the pot and shift into the oven.
Bake for around 2¼ hours, flipping the shanks after every 45 minutes.
Take off the lid and bake for around 20 more minutes.
Take off the pot from the oven and discard the bay leaves.
Enjoy right away.

INGREDIENTS REQUIRED:

- Olive oil – 2 tbsp. (30 ml)
- Lamb shanks – 2 (12-oz.) (340-g)
- Medium-sized onion – ½, cut up
- Garlic cloves – 3, minced
- Dried rosemary – ½ tsp.
- Dried thyme – ½ tsp.
- Ground cumin – 1 tsp.
- Paprika – 1 tsp.
- Red wine – 1 C. (240 ml)
- Salt and ground black pepper – as desired
- Chicken broth – 2½ C. (600 ml)
- Bay leaves – 2

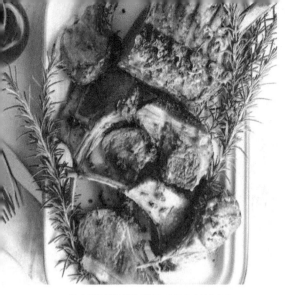

Garlicky Rack of Lamb

Prep period: 15 mins.
Cook period: 50 mins.
Serves: 6

Per Serving: Calories 573, Fat 33.5g
Carbs 1.6g, Protein 64g

INGREDIENTS REQUIRED:

- Olive oil – ½ C. plus 1 tbsp. (135 ml), divided
- Garlic cloves – 6, crushed
- Fresh thyme sprig – 1, cut up
- Fresh rosemary sprig – 1, cut up
- Red pepper flakes – ½ tsp., crushed
- Lamb racks – 2 (1½-lb.) (680-g), frenched
- Salt and ground black pepper – as desired

PROCEDURE:

1. Put ½ C. of oil, garlic, fresh herbs, and red pepper flakes int a large baking pan and blend thoroughly.
2. Put in lamb racks and coat with marinade generously.
3. Cover and put in your fridge fo at least 6 hours, flipping from time to time.
4. Take it out of the fridge and set the baking tray aside at room temperature for 1 hour before cooking.
5. For preheating: set your oven a 275 °F (140 °C).
6. Take the lamb racks out of the baking pan, reserving the marinade.
7. Sprinkle each lamb rack with s and pepper.
8. Sizzle remnant oil into a large cast-iron pot on a burner at medium-high heat.
9. Sear the lamb shanks for 3-4 minutes.

ROCEDURE:

With a slotted spoon, place the lamb racks onto a plate.
Put the reserved marinade into the pan.
Cook for 2 minutes.
Take it off the burner and set it aside to cool slightly.
Lay out the racks into the pan, meat-side down, with the bones upright.
Place the wok into the oven and bake for around 30-40 minutes, basting with the pot juices after every 5 minutes.
Take it out of the oven and set it aside for around 20 minutes before carving.
Cut the lamb racks into individual chops and enjoy.

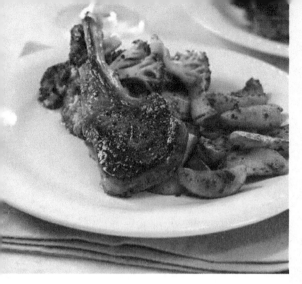

Spicy Lamb Chops

Prep period: 10 mins.
Cook period: 6 mins.
Serves: 4

Per Serving: Calories 467, Fat 20.7
Carbs 2.4g, Protein 64.4g

INGREDIENTS REQUIRED:

- Garlic cloves – 4, peeled
- Salt – as desired
- Ground cumin – 2 tsp.
- Ground coriander – 1 tsp.
- Ground cinnamon – ½ tsp.
- Ground ginger – ½ tsp.
- Ground black pepper – as desired
- Lamb chops – 8 (4-oz.) (110-g), trimmed
- Olive oil – 1 tbsp. (15 ml)
- Lemon juice – 1 tbsp. (15 ml), freshly squeezed

PROCEDURE:

1. Place the garlic cloves onto a chopping board and sprinkle with some salt.
2. With a knife, crush the garlic t form a paste.
3. Place the garlic paste into a basin.
4. Put in spices and pepper and blend thoroughly.
5. With a sharp knife, make 3-4 cuts on both sides of the chop
6. Rub the chops with the garlic mixture generously.
7. Sizzle oil into a large-sized cast-iron wok on the burner a around medium heat.
8. Cook the chops for around 3 minutes per side.
9. Drizzle with lemon juice and enjoy right away.

Rosemary Beef Tenderloin

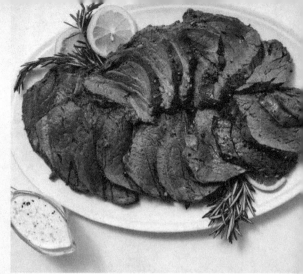

Prep period: 10 mins.
Cook period: 50 mins.
Serves: 10

er Serving: Calories 295, Fat 13.9g,
Carbs 0.6g, Protein 39.5g

PROCEDURE:

For preheating: set your oven at 425 ºF (220 ºC).
Spray a large, shallow roasting pan with baking spray.
Lay out the beef tenderloin into the roasting pan.
Rub the roast with garlic, rosemary, salt, and pepper, and drizzle with oil.
Roast for around 45-50 minutes. Take it out of the oven and place the roast onto a chopping board for around 10 minutes.
Cut the beef tenderloin into serving portions and enjoy.

INGREDIENTS REQUIRED:

- Olive oil baking spray
- Center-cut beef tenderloin – 1 (3-lb.) (1360-g)
- Garlic cloves – 4, minced
- Fresh rosemary – 2 tbsp., minced
- Salt and ground black pepper – as desired
- Olive oil – 1 tbsp. (15 ml)

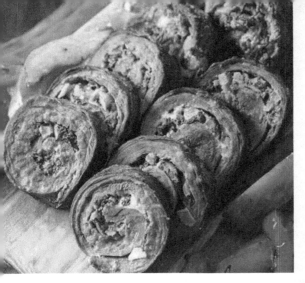

Stuffed Steak

Prep period: 15 mins.
Cook period: 35 mins.
Serves: 6

Per Serving: Calories 395, Fat 18.2
Carbs 7.3g, Protein 48.4g

INGREDIENTS REQUIRED:

- Dried oregano – 2 tsp.
- Lemon juice – 1/3 C. (90 ml) freshly squeezed
- Olive oil – 2 tbsp. (30 ml)
- Beef flank steak – 1 (2-lb.) (910-g), pounded into ½-inch thickness.
- Frozen chopped spinach – 1 C. (30 g)
- Olive tapenade – 1/3 C. (100 g)
- Feta cheese – ¼ C. (30 g), crumbled
- Fresh cherry tomatoes – 4 C. (600 g)
- Salt – as desired

PROCEDURE:

1. Put the oregano, lemon juice, and oil into a large baking pan and stir thoroughly.
2. Put in steak and coat generous with the marinade.
3. Put into your fridge to marina for around 4 hours, flipping from time to time.
4. For preheating: set your oven 425 °F (220 °C).
5. Line a shallow baking pan wit parchment paper.
6. Take the steak out of the bakir pan, reserving the remnant marinade into a basin.
7. Cover the basin of marinade a reserve it in your fridge.
8. Thaw the frozen spinach and then squeeze to remove exces water. Set it aside.
9. Lay out the steak on a choppir board.
10. Place the tapenade onto the steak and top with the spinacl followed by the feta cheese.

·······································

·······································

·······································

·······································

·······································

PROCEDURE:

·······································

1. Carefully roll the steak tightly to form a log.
·······································
2. With 6 kitchen string pieces, tie the log at 6 places.
·······································
3. Carefully cut the log between strings into 6 equal pieces, leaving the string in place.
·······································
4. Put the reserved marinade, tomatoes, and salt into a basin and toss to incorporate.
·······································
5. Lay out the log pieces onto the baking pan cut-side up.
·······································
6. Lay out the tomatoes around the pinwheels.
·······································
. Bake for around 25-35 minutes.
·······································
8. Take the baking pan of steak out of the oven and set it aside for around 5 minutes before enjoying.
·······································

·······································

·······································

·······································

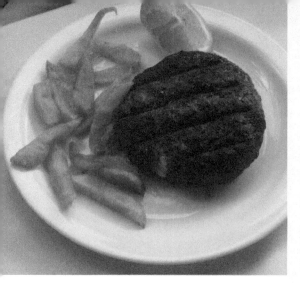

Beef Bifteki

Prep period: 15 mins.
Cook period: 20 mins.
Serves: 4

Per Serving: Calories 369, Fat 15.8g
Carbs 1.8g, Protein 51.6g

INGREDIENTS REQUIRED:

- Olive oil baking spray
- Ground beef – 1 1/3 lb. (650 g)
- Plain Greek yogurt – 1 tbsp. (15 g)
- Dried thyme – 2 tsp.
- Salt and ground black pepper – as desired
- Feta cheese – 4 oz. (110 g), cut into 4 slices

PROCEDURE:

1. For preheating: set your grill fc indirect heat.
2. Spray the grill grate with bakin spray.
3. Put the ground beef and remnant ingredients except for feta into a large basin and stir
4. to incorporate thoroughly.
5. Make 8 patties from the mixtu
6. Place 1 cheese slice between tw patties and press slightly to sea the edges.
7. Repeat with remnant beef patt and cheese slices.
8. Lay out the patties onto the gri and cover with its lid.
9. Cook for around 15-20 minute
10. Enjoy right away.

Pistachio-Crusted Pork Tenderloin

Prep period: 15 mins.

Cook period: 22 mins.

Serves: 4

Per Serving: Calories 258, Fat 9.8g, Carbs 11.8g, Protein 30.8g

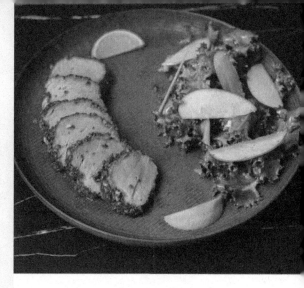

PROCEDURE:

For preheating: lay out a rack in the center of the oven.

Set your oven at 450 ºF (230 ºC).

Put the pistachios and garlic into an electric food processor and process to cut up finely.

Rub the pork tenderloin with salt and pepper.

Sizzle oil into a large-sized cast-iron wok on the burner at around medium-high heat.

Cook the pork for around 4-6 minutes.

Take off the wok from the burner.

Coat the top of the pork with orange marmalade, followed by the pistachio mixture.

With your hands, gently press the pistachio mixture into the meat.

Roast for around 12-16 minutes.

Take out of the oven and place the pork tenderloin onto a chopping board for around 5 minutes.

Cut the pork tenderloin into serving portions and enjoy.

INGREDIENTS REQUIRED:

- Pistachios – 1/3 C. (50 g), shelled and toasted
- Garlic cloves – 2, peeled
- Pork tenderloin – 1 lb. (455 g), trimmed
- Salt and ground black pepper – as desired
- Olive oil – 1 tbsp. (15 ml)
- Orange marmalade – 3 tbsp. (60 g)

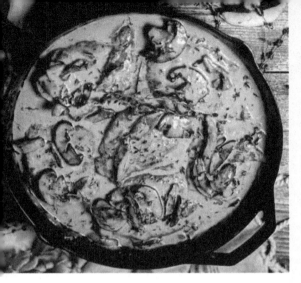

Pork Chops with Mushroom Sauce

Prep period: 15 mins.

Cook period: 25 mins.

Serves: 4

Per Serving: Calories 415, Fat 21.8g
Carbs 6.9g, Protein 26.4g

INGREDIENTS REQUIRED:

- Boneless pork chops – 4
- Paprika – ½ tsp.
- Salt and ground black pepper – as desired
- Olive oil – 2 tsp. (10 ml)
- Unsalted butter – 3 tbsp. (40 g), divided
- Fresh mushrooms – 8 oz. (226 g), sliced
- Medium-sized onion – ½, finely cut up
- Garlic cloves – 2, minced
- All-purpose flour – 1 tbsp. (8 g)
- Chicken broth – 1½ C. (30 ml)
- Heavy cream – 1/3 C. (90 g)
- Hot sauce – 1 tsp. (5 g)
- Fresh parsley – 2 tbsp., cut up

PROCEDURE:

1. Rub the pork chops with paprika, sa and pepper.
2. Sizzle 1 tbsp. of butter and oil into a large pot and on the burner at medium-high heat.
3. Sear the chops for around 3-4 minut per side.
4. With a slotted spoon, shift the chops onto a plate and cover with a piece o heavy-duty foil to keep them warm.
5. Sizzle 1 tbsp. of the remnant butter i the same pot on the burner at mediu heat.
6. Cook the mushrooms for around 2 minutes, stirring frequently.
7. Put in remnant butter, onions, salt, a pepper and blend.
8. Cook for around 3-4 minutes, stirrin frequently.
9. Put in the garlic and blend.
10. Cook for around 1 minute, stirring frequently.
11. Put in flour and stir vigorously for a least 30 seconds.
12. Put in broth, cream, hot sauce, salt, pepper, and stir.
13. Cook for around 2 minutes, stirring the time.
14. Stir in pork chops and turn the heat around low.
15. Cook with the cover for around 5-8 minutes.
16. Enjoy right away with the garnishin parsley.

Sausage with Apples

Prep period: 10 mins.
Cook period: 30 mins.
Serves: 6

er Serving: Calories 227, Fat 12.2g,
Carbs 8g, Protein 19.8g

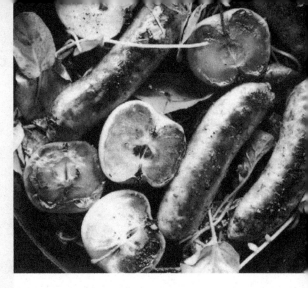

PROCEDURE:

Sizzle oil into a large-sized cast-iron wok on the burner at medium-high heat.
Place the apples into the wok cut side down.
Cook for around 5-8 minutes, flipping from time to time.
Put in sausages and cook for around 10-12 minutes, flipping from time to time.
Put in wine and vinegar and stir.
Cook the mixture until boiling.
Turn the heat to low.
Cook for 4 minutes and stir.
Put in watercress, salt, and pepper.
Cook for 1-2 minutes.
Enjoy right away.

INGREDIENTS REQUIRED:

- Olive oil – 1 tbsp. (15 ml)
- Apples – 1 lb. (455 g), halved through stem ends
- Sweet Italian sausages – 1½ lb. (680 g), pricked
- Dry white wine – ¼ C. (60 ml)
- White wine vinegar – 2 tbsp. (30 ml)
- Watercress – 8 C. (280 g), trimmed
- Salt and ground black pepper – as desired

NOTES

FISH & SEAFOOD RECIPES

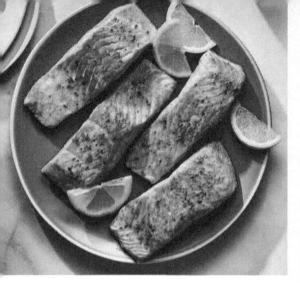

Spicy Salmon

Prep period: 10 mins.
Cook period: 8 mins.
Serves: 4

Per Serving: Calories 368, Fat 24.4g
Carbs 2.8g, Protein 34g

INGREDIENTS REQUIRED:

- Ground cumin – 2 tsp.
- Red chili powder – 2 tsp.
- Paprika – 2 tsp.
- Garlic cloves – 4, minced
- Salt and ground black pepper – as desired
- Skinless salmon fillets – 4 (6-oz.) (150-g)
- Unsalted butter – 2 tbsp. (30 g)

PROCEDURE:

1. Put the spices into a small-size basin and blend thoroughly.
2. Coat the salmon fillets with a spice mixture.
3. Sizzle butter into a cast-iron w on the burner at medium-high heat.
4. Cook the salmon fillets for 3 minutes.
5. Flip the salmon fillets.
6. Cook for 4-5 minutes.
7. Enjoy right away.

Parmesan Tilapia

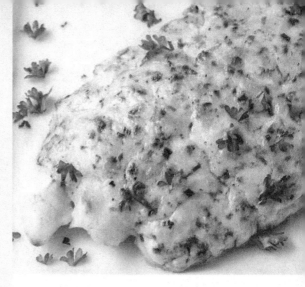

Prep period: 10 mins.
Cook period: 5 mins.
Serves: 4

Per Serving: Calories 185, Fat 9.8g,
Carbs 1.4g, Protein 23.2g

PROCEDURE:

For preheating: set your oven to broiler.
Spray a broiler pan with baking spray.
Put the cheese and remnant ingredients except tilapia fillets into a large-sized basin and blend to incorporate. Set it aside.
Lay out the fillets onto the broiler pan.
Broil the fillets for around 2-3 minutes.
Take off the broiler pan from the oven and top the fillets with the cheese mixture.
Broil for around 2 minutes further.
Enjoy right away.

INGREDIENTS REQUIRED:

- Olive oil baking spray
- Parmesan cheese – ½ C. (55 g), grated
- Mayonnaise – 3 tbsp. (25 g)
- Unsalted butter –¼ C. (55 g), softened
- Lemon juice – 2 tbsp. (30 ml), freshly squeezed
- Dried thyme – ½ tsp. , crushed
- Salt and ground black pepper – as desired
- Tilapia fillets – 4 (4-oz.) (110-g)

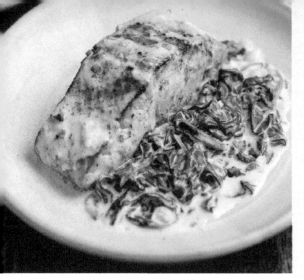

Salmon in Creamy Spinach Sauce

Prep period: 15 mins.
Cook period: 10 mins.
Serves: 4

Per Serving: Calories 610, Fat 51g, Carbs 5.8g, Protein 30.1g

INGREDIENTS REQUIRED:

- Lemon pepper seasoning – ½ tsp.
- Dried thyme – 1 tsp.
- Dried parsley – 1 tsp.
- Boneless salmon fillets – 4 (5-oz.) (140-g)
- Lemon juice – 5 tbsp. (75 ml), freshly squeezed and divided
- Unsalted butter – 10 tbsp. (140 g), divided
- Shallot – 1 minced
- White wine – 5 tbsp. (75 ml), divided
- White wine vinegar – 1 tbsp. (15 ml)
- Half-and-half – 1 C. (240 g)
- Fresh spinach – 3 C. (90 g), cut up
- Salt and ground white pepper – as desired

PROCEDURE:

1. Put the lemon pepper seasonin and dried herbs into a small basin and stir to incorporate.
2. Put the salmon fillets into a shallow dish and rub with 3 tb of lemon juice.
3. Rub the non-skin side with the herb mixture. Set it aside.
4. Sizzle 2 tbsp. of butter into a w on the burner at medium heat.
5. Place salmon in the wok, herb side down.
6. Cook for around 1-2 minutes.
7. Shift the salmon fillets onto a plate, herb side up.
8. Put 1 tbsp. of wine in the wok and scrape up the browned bit from the bottom.
9. Place the salmon fillets into th wok, herb side up.
10. Cook for around 8 minutes.
11. In the meantime, sizzle 2 tbsp. butter into a wok on a burner medium heat.

PROCEDURE:

2. Cook the shallot for around 2 minutes.
3. Put in remnant lemon juice, remnant wine, and vinegar and stir.
4. Cook for around 2-3 minutes.
5. Put in half-and-half spinach, salt, and white pepper and blend.
6. Cook for 2-3 minutes.
7. Put in remnant butter and whisk to incorporate thoroughly.
8. Take it off the burner and set it aside with the cover on to keep it warm.
9. Place the salmon fillets onto serving plates.
10. Top with pan sauce and enjoy.

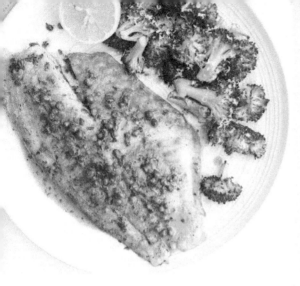

Tilapia Piccata

Prep period: 10 mins.

Cook period: 8 mins.

Serves: 4

Per Serving: Calories 206, Fat 8.7g
Carbs 0.9g, Protein 31.9g

INGREDIENTS REQUIRED:

- Olive oil baking spray
- Lemon juice – 3 tbsp. (45 ml), freshly squeezed
- Olive oil – 2 tbsp. (30 ml)
- Garlic cloves – 2, minced
- Lemon zest – ½ tsp., grated
- Capers – 1 tbsp. (8 g), liquid removed
- Fresh basil – 2 tbsp., minced and divided
- Tilapia fillets – 4 (6-oz.) (150-g)
- Salt and ground black pepper – as desired

PROCEDURE:

1. For preheating: lay out a rack about 4 inches from the heatir element.
2. Set your oven to broiler.
3. Spray a broiler pan with bakir spray.
4. Put the lemon juice, oil, garlic and lemon zest into a small basin and whisk to incorporat thoroughly.
5. Put in capers and 2 tbsp. of ba and blend to incorporate.
6. Reserve 2 tbsp. of the mixture into a small basin.
7. Coat the fish fillets with remn capers mixture and sprinkle v salt and pepper.
8. Place the tilapia fillets onto th broiler pan and broil for 3-4 minutes per side.
9. Take out of the oven and plac the fish fillets onto serving plates.
10. Drizzle with reserved capers mixture and enjoy with the garnishing of remnant basil.

Cod, Olives & Tomato Bake

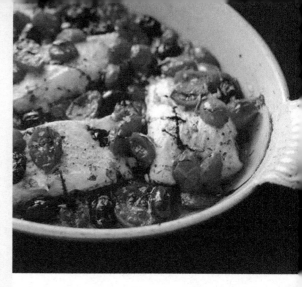

Prep period: 15 mins.
Cook period: 20 mins.
Serves: 4

er Serving: Calories 468, Fat 20.4g,
Carbs 7.3g, Protein 52.1g

PROCEDURE:

For preheating: set your oven at 350 ºF (175 ºC).
Put the onion, tomato, olives, capers, oil, lemon juice, salt, and pepper into a basin and blend thoroughly.
Rub the cod fillets with Greek seasoning.
Place the cod fillets in a baking pan.
Top the fillets with the tomato mixture.
Bake for around 15-20 minutes.
Enjoy right away.

INGREDIENTS REQUIRED:

- Medium-sized onion – 1, cut up
- Cherry tomatoes – 2 C. (300 g), halved
- Kalamata olives – 1 (5-oz.) (140-g) jar, pitted
- Capers – ¼ C. (30 g)
- Olive oil – ¼ C. (60 ml)
- Lemon juice – 1 tbsp. (15 ml), freshly squeezed
- Salt and ground black pepper – as desired
- Tuna fillets – 4 (6-oz.) (150-g)
- Greek seasoning – 2 tsp.

Shrimp Scampi

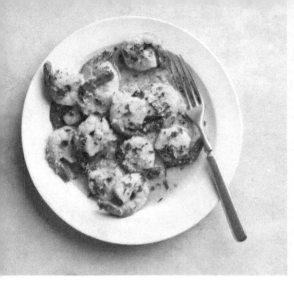

Prep period: 15 mins.
Cook period: 15 mins.
Serves: 4

Per Serving: Calories 626, Fat 38.1g
Carbs 18.4g, Protein 7.4g

INGREDIENTS REQUIRED:

- Unsalted butter – ½ C. plus 1 tbsp. (140 g), divided
- Garlic cloves – 4, minced
- White wine – 1 C. (240 ml)
- Shrimp – 1 lb. (455 g), peeled and deveined
- Italian breadcrumbs – ½ C. (75 g)

PROCEDURE:

1. For preheating: set your oven at 350 °F (175 °C).
2. Sizzle ½ C. of butter into a small-sized pot on a burner at medium heat.
3. Cook the garlic for around 30 seconds.
4. Put in white wine and stir.
5. Cook for around 1-2 minutes.
6. Put the remnant butter into a small-sized microwave-safe dish and microwave until melted.
7. Take out of the microwave and stir in breadcrumbs to incorporate thoroughly.
8. Place shrimp into a baking pan and top with wine mixture, followed by the buttered breadcrumbs.
9. Bake for around 10-12 minutes.
10. Enjoy right away.

Shrimp in Tomato Sauce

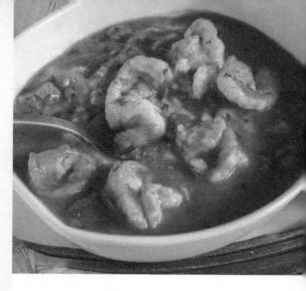

Prep period: 15 mins.

Cook period: 18 mins.

Serves: 6

Per Serving: Calories 289, Fat 16g, Carbs 7g, Protein 27.1g

PROCEDURE:

Sizzle oil into a wok on the burner at medium heat.
Cook the onion for 4-5 minutes.
Put in red pepper and garlic and stir.
Cook for 4-5 minutes.
Put in shrimp and tomatoes and stir.
Cook for 2 minutes.
Put in wine and broth and stir.
Cook for 4-5 minutes.
Stir in lemon juice, salt, and pepper, and take off from the burner.
Garnish with parsley, and enjoy right away.

INGREDIENTS REQUIRED:

- Olive oil – ¼ C. (60 ml)
- Onions – ¼ C. (30 g), cut up
- Roasted red peppers – ¼ C. (40 g), cut up
- Garlic clove – 1, minced
- Shrimp – 1½ lb. (680 g), peeled and deveined
- Diced tomatoes – 1 (14-oz.) (400-g) can
- Red wine – ¼ C. (60 ml)
- Chicken broth – ¾ C. (180 ml)
- Lemon juice – 2 tbsp. (30 ml), freshly squeezed
- Salt and ground black pepper – as desired
- Fresh parsley – ¼ C., cut up

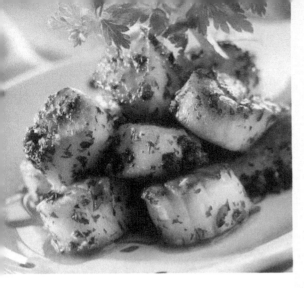

Buttered Scallops

Prep period: 10 mins.
Cook period: 7 mins.
Serves: 2

Per Serving: Calories 273, Fat 19.5g
Carbs 3.7g, Protein 20.5g

INGREDIENTS REQUIRED:

- Large-sized sea scallops – 8, side muscle removed
- Salt and ground black pepper – as desired
- Olive oil – 1 tbsp. (15 ml)
- Unsalted butter – 2 tbsp. (30 g)
- Garlic cloves – 2, minced
- Fresh parsley – 2 tbsp., minced
- Lemon juice – 1 tbsp. (15 ml), freshly squeezed

PROCEDURE:

1. Sprinkle the scallops with salt and pepper.
2. Sizzle oil into a cast-iron wok the burner at medium-high he
3. Sear the scallops for 2 minutes per side.
4. With a slotted spoon, place the scallops onto a plate.
5. Put the butter, garlic, parsley, and lemon juice in the same w and blend it.
6. Cook for around 1-2 minutes, stirring from time to time.
7. Put in cooked scallops and blend.
8. Cook for around 1 minute.
9. Enjoy right away.

Mussels in Tomato Sauce

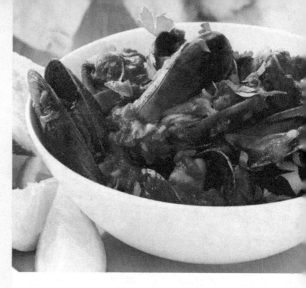

Prep period: 15 mins.
Cook period: 18 mins.
Serves: 6

Per Serving: Calories 244, Fat 6g,
Carbs 14.3g, Protein 19.1g

PROCEDURE:

Sizzle oil into a large-sized wok on the burner at medium heat.
Cook the celery, onion, and garlic for around 5 minutes.
Put in tomato, honey, and red pepper flakes and blend.
Cook for 10 minutes.
In the meantime, put the mussels and wine into a large pot on a burner at medium heat.
Cook the mixture until boiling.
Cook with the cover on for 10 minutes.
Shift the mussel mixture into the tomato mixture and stir to incorporate.
Stir in salt and pepper and take off the burner.
Enjoy right away with the garnishing of basil.

INGREDIENTS REQUIRED:

- Olive oil – 1 tbsp. (15 ml)
- Celery stalks – 2, cut up
- Medium-sized onion – 1, cut up
- Garlic cloves – 4, minced
- Dried oregano – ½ tsp., crushed
- Diced tomatoes – 1 (15-oz.) (425-g) can
- Honey – 1 tbsp.
- Red pepper flakes – 1 tsp., crushed
- Mussels – 2 lb. (910 g), cleaned
- White wine – 2 C. (480 ml)
- Salt and ground black pepper – as desired
- Fresh basil – ¼ C. (5 g), cut up

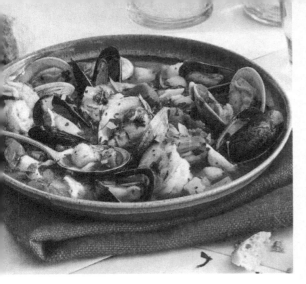

Seafood & Tomato Stew

Prep period: 20 mins.
Cook period: 25 mins.
Serves: 4

Per Serving: Calories 313, Fat 7.8g
Carbs 11.6g, Protein 44.3g

INGREDIENTS REQUIRED:

- Olive oil – 2 tbsp. (30 ml)
- Medium-sized onion – 1, finely cut up
- Garlic cloves – 2, minced
- Red pepper flakes – ¼ tsp., crushed
- Plum tomatoes – ½ lb. (220 g), cut up
- White wine – 1/3 C. (90 ml)
- Clam juice – 1 C. (240 ml)
- Tomato paste – 1 tbsp. (20 g)
- Salt – as desired
- Snapper fillets – 1 lb. (455 g), cubed into 1-inch size
- Shrimp – 1 lb. (455 g), peeled and deveined
- Sea scallops – ½ lb. (226 g), side muscle removed
- Fresh parsley – ¼ C. (5 g), minced
- Lemon zest – 1 tsp., grated finely

PROCEDURE:

1. Sizzle oil into a large-sized Dut oven on the burner at medium heat.
2. Cook the onion for 3-4 minute
3. Put in garlic and red pepper fla and blend.
4. Cook for 1 minute.
5. Put in tomatoes and blend.
6. Cook for 2 minutes.
7. Put in wine, clam juice, tomato paste, and salt and blend.
8. Cook the mixture until boiling
9. Turn the heat to low.
10. Cook with the cover on for 10 minutes.
11. Put in seafood and stir.
12. Cook with the cover on for 6-8 minutes.
13. Blend in parsley and take off th burner.
14. Enjoy right away with the garnishing of lemon zest.

DESSERT RECIPES

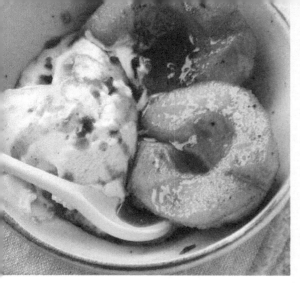

Maple Baked Pears

Prep period: 10 mins.
Cook period: 25 mins.
Serves: 4

Per Serving: Calories Calories 227,
Fat 0.4g, Carbs 58.5g, Protein 0.8g

INGREDIENTS REQUIRED:

- Anjou pears – 4, halved and cored
- Ground cinnamon – ¼ tsp.
- Maple syrup – ½ C. (150 g)
- Vanilla extract – 1 tsp. (5 ml)

PROCEDURE:

1. For preheating: set your oven a 375 ºF (190 ºC).
2. Line a baking tray with bakery paper.
3. Carefully cut a small sliver off the underside of each pear half
4. Place the pear halves onto the baking tray, cut side upwards, and sprinkle with cinnamon.
5. Put the maple syrup and vanill extract into a small basin and whisk thoroughly.
6. Reserve about 2 tbsp. of the maple syrup mixture.
7. Place the remnant maple syrup mixture over the pears.
8. Bake for around 25 minutes.
9. Take it out of the oven and immediately drizzle it with the reserved maple syrup mixture.
10. Enjoy moderately hot.

Fruity Yogurt Parfait

Prep period: 10 mins.

Cook period: 10 mins.

Serves: 4

Per Serving: Calories 269, Fat 4.9g, Carbs 48.5g, Protein 9.5g

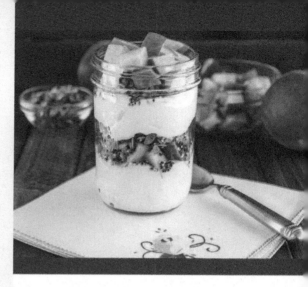

PROCEDURE:

Put the yogurt and honey into a medium glass basin and stir to incorporate thoroughly.

Put the remaining ingredients, except for almonds, into a pot on the burner at around medium heat.

Cook for around 8-10 minutes, stirring from time to time.

Take it off the burner and set it aside at room temperature to cool.

Divide half of the yogurt mixture into 4 tall serving glasses.

Divide the fruit mixture over yogurt and top each with the remnant yogurt.

Garnish with almonds and enjoy.

INGREDIENTS REQUIRED:

- Plain Greek yogurt – 2 C. (500 g)
- Honey – ¼ C. (75 g)
- Water – ¼ C. (60 ml)
- White sugar – 2 tbsp. (25 g)
- Lime zest – ½ tsp. (1 g), finely grated
- Ground cinnamon – ¼ tsp.
- Vanilla extract – ¼ tsp.
- Peaches – 2, pitted and quartered
- Plums – 4, pitted and quartered
- Almonds – ¼ C. (25 g), toasted and cut up

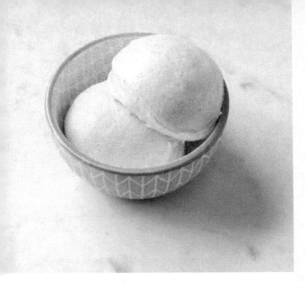

Ricotta Gelato

Prep period: 10 mins.

Cook period: 10 mins.

Serves: 8

Per Serving: Calories 89, Fat 1.5g,
Carbs 8.7g, Protein 7g

INGREDIENTS REQUIRED:

- Fresh ricotta cheese – 2 C. (440 g)
- Whole milk – 2 C. (480 ml)
- Ground cinnamon – ¼ tsp.
- Ground nutmeg – 1 pinch
- White sugar – 1 C. (200 g)
- Large-sized egg yolks – 5
- Heavy cream – 1 C. (240 g)

PROCEDURE:

1. Line a sieve with cheesecloth a
   arrange over a basin.
2. Place the ricotta cheese into th
   sieve.
3. Put the basin of ricotta cheese
   into your fridge overnight to
   drain.
4. Put the milk, cinnamon, and
   nutmeg into a medium pot on
   burner at medium-low heat.
5. Cook the mixture until boiling
6. Take off the pot of milk mixtur
   from the burner and set it asid
7. Put the sugar and egg yolks int
   a basin and whisk them with a
   electric mixer to form a thick
   and pale yellow mixture.
8. Put in half of the warm
   milk mixture and whisk to
   incorporate thoroughly.
9. Place the mixture in the pot w
   the remnant milk mixture.
10. Return the pot to the burner a

···

···

···

···

···

PROCEDURE:

···

low heat.
. Cook until the mixture becomes
thick, stirring all the time.
. Take off the pot from the burner
and immediately stir in heavy
cream.
. Place a fine sieve over a basin.
. Strain the milk mixture into the
basin and cool over an ice bath.
. Now, with the electric mixer, whisk
the mixture thoroughly.
Pour the mixture into an ice cream
maker and freeze according to the
manufacturer's directions.
Now, place the mixture into a
sealable container and freeze until
set thoroughly before enjoying.

···

···

···

···

···

···

···

···

···

···

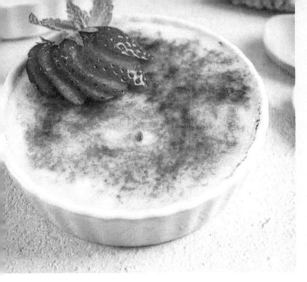

Strawberry Crème Brûlée

Prep period: 20 mins.
Cook period: 1 hr. 10 mins.
Serves: 8

Per Serving: Calories 296, Fat 14.5
Carbs 32g, Protein 11.1g

INGREDIENTS REQUIRED:

- Fresh strawberries – 2¼ C. (280 g), hulled and cut up
- White sugar – ½ C. (100 g)
- Heavy cream – 2 C. (480 g)
- Strawberry milk – 2 C. (480 ml)
- Vanilla extract – 2 tsp.
- Egg yolks – 6
- Ground sugar – ½ C. (65 g)

PROCEDURE:

1. For preheating: set your oven a 325 ºF (165 ºC).
2. Put the strawberries into a pot and sprinkle with 1 tbsp. of sugar.
3. Place the pot on the burner at low heat.
4. Cook the mixture until boiling
5. Cook for around 5-8 minutes.
6. Take off the burner and set it aside to cool slightly.
7. Put the cream and strawberry milk in the pot of strawberry sauce and whisk to incorporat thoroughly.
8. Place the pot of sauce mixture on the burner at medium heat
9. Cook until just scalded but no boiling.
10. Take off from the burner and it aside.
11. Put the eggs and remnant sug in a whisk to form a thick and pale texture.

PROCEDURE:

2. Put in vanilla extract and blend thoroughly.
3. Slowly pour the warmed cream mixture into the egg mixture to incorporate thoroughly.
4. Place the mixture into 8 shallow ramekins.
5. Place the ramekins into a baking pan.
6. Put hot water into the baking pan, about 1 inch up the sides of the ramekins.
7. Bake for around 45-60 minutes.
8. Take the baking pan of ramekins out of the oven and let them cool slightly.
9. Put the ramekins into your fridge for at least 4 hours.
. Just before enjoying, sprinkle the ramekins with ground Erythritol.
. Holding a kitchen torch about 4-5-inch from the top, caramelize the Erythritol for around 2 minutes.
. Set them aside for 5 minutes before enjoying them.

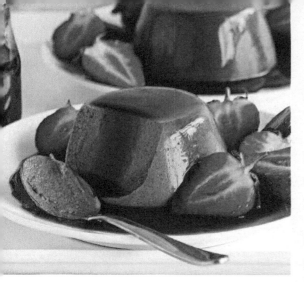

Chocolate Pana Cotta

Prep period: 10 mins.
Cook period: 5 mins.
Serves: 4

Per Serving: Calories 136, Fat 12.1g, Carbs 5.8g, Protein 4.4g

INGREDIENTS REQUIRED:

- Unsweetened almond milk – 1½ C. (360 ml), divided
- Unflavored gelatin powder – 1 tbsp. (9 g)
- Unsweetened coconut milk – 1 C. (240 ml)
- White sugar – 1/3 C. (75 g)
- Cocoa powder – 3 tbsp. (25 g)
- Instant coffee granules – 2 tsp. (6 g)
- Liquid stevia – 6 drops

PROCEDURE:

1. Put ½ C. of almond milk into a large-sized basin and sprinkle with gelatin.
2. Set it aside until soaked.
3. Put the remnant almond milk, coconut milk, sugar, cocoa powder, coffee granules, and stevia into a pot on a burner at medium heat.
4. Cook the mixture until boiling stirring all the time.
5. Take off from the burner.
6. Put the gelatin mixture and hot milk mixture into an electric blender and process to form a smooth mixture.
7. Place the mixture into serving glasses and set them aside to cool thoroughly.
8. With plastic wrap, cover each glass and put them into your fridge for around 3-4 hours before enjoying.

Cream Cheese Flan

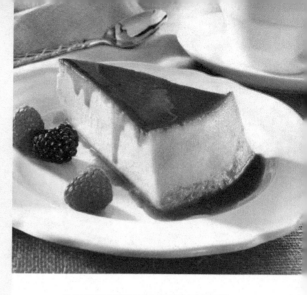

Prep period: 15 mins.
Cook period: 1 hr. 5 mins.
Serves: 8

er Serving: Calories 320, Fat 24.1g, Carbs 20.7g, Protein 6.7g

PROCEDURE:

For preheating: set your oven at 350 ºF (175 ºC).

Spray an 8-inch cake pan with baking spray.

For the caramel: put ½ C. of the sugar, 2 tbsp. of water and 1 tsp. of vanilla extract into a heavy-bottomed pot on a burner at medium-low heat.

Cook until the sweetener is melted thoroughly, stirring all the time.

Take off the pot of caramel from the burner and place the caramel in the bottom of the cake pan.

Put the remnant sugar, vanilla extract, heavy cream, cream cheese, eggs, and salt into an electric blender and process to form a smooth mixture.

Place the cream cheese mixture over the caramel.

Place the cake pan into a large roasting pan.

Put hot water into the roasting pan about 1 inch up the sides of the cake pan.

Bake for around 1 hour.

Take out of the oven and place the cake pan in a water bath to cool thoroughly.

Put it into your fridge for around 4-5 hours before enjoying it.

INGREDIENTS REQUIRED:

- Olive oil baking spray
- White sugar – ¾ C. (150 g), divided
- Water – 3 tbsp. (45 ml), divided
- Vanilla extract – 2 tsp. (10 ml), divided
- Large-sized eggs – 5
- Heavy cream – 2 C. (480 g)
- Cream cheese – 8 oz. (220 g), softened
- Salt – ¼ tsp.

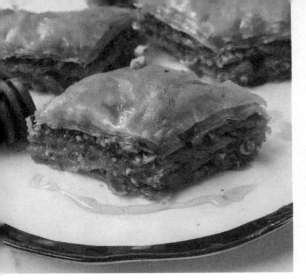

Baklava

Prep period: 15 mins.

Cook period: 50 mins.

Serves: 18

Per Serving: Calories 392, Fat 25.9

Carbs 37.9g, Protein 5.9g

INGREDIENTS REQUIRED:

- Olive oil baking spray
- Mixed nuts (pistachios, almonds, walnuts) – 1 lb. (455 g), cut up
- Ground cinnamon – 1 tsp.
- Filo dough – 1 (16-oz.) (455-g) package
- Unsalted butter – 1 C. (225 g) liquefied
- White sugar – 1 C. (200 g)
- Water – 1 C. (240 ml)
- Honey – ½ C. (150 g)
- Vanilla extract – 1 tsp. (5 ml)

PROCEDURE:

1. For preheating: set your oven at 3 ᵒF (175 ᵒC).
2. Spray a 9x13-inch baking pan wit baking spray.
3. Put the nuts and cinnamon into a basin and toss to incorporate thoroughly. Set it aside.
4. Unroll the filo dough and cut it ir half.
5. Lay out 2 dough sheets into the baking pan and coat with some butter.
6. Repeat with 8 dough sheets in lay and sprinkle with 2-- 3 tbsp. of n mixture.
7. Repeat with remnant dough shee butter, and nuts.
8. Cut into diamond shapes all the v to the bottom of the baking pan.
9. Bake for around 50 minutes.
10. In the meantime, for the sauce: c the sugar and water in a pot unti melted, stirring all the time.
11. Put in honey and vanilla extract blend.
12. Cook for around 20 minutes.
13. Take the baklava from out of the oven and immediately place the sauce on top.
14. Set it aside to cool before enjoyir

Fig Cake

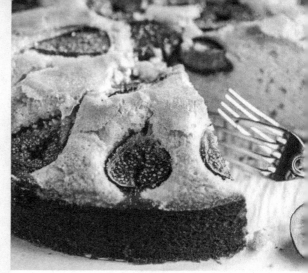

Prep period: 15 mins.

Cook period: 55 mins.

Serves: 8

er Serving: Calories 365, Fat 14.1g,
Carbs 58.1g, Protein 5.6g

PROCEDURE:

For preheating: lay out a rack in the center portion of the oven.
Set your oven at 350 ºF (175 ºC).
Spray a 9-inch springform pan with baking spray and then dust it with flour lightly.
Sift together the flour, baking powder, and salt into a large-sized basin.
Put in the lemon zest and blend thoroughly.
Put sugar and eggs into a separate bowl and, with a hand blender, whisk to form a thick and pale yellow mixture.
Put in milk, oil, butter, and vanilla extract and whisk to incorporate thoroughly.
Put in flour mixture, and stir with a wooden spoon to incorporate thoroughly.
Set it aside for around 10 minutes.
Put about ¾ of the figs in the basin of flour mixture and gently blend to incorporate.
Place the mixture into the cake pan.
Bake for 15 minutes.
Take it out of the oven and top the cake with the remnant figs.
Bake for around 35-40 minutes.

INGREDIENTS REQUIRED:

- Olive oil baking spray
- Unbleached all-purpose flour – 1½ C. (195 g) plus more for dusting
- Baking powder – ¾ tsp.
- Salt – 1 pinch
- Lemon zest – 1 tsp. (2 g), finely grated
- White sugar – 2/3 C. (145 g)
- Large-sized eggs – 2
- Whole milk – 1/3 C. (90 ml)
- Olive oil – ¼ C. (60 ml)
- Unsalted butter – ¼ C. (55 g) liquefied
- Vanilla extract – ½ tsp.
- Fresh figs – 10 oz. (280 g), cut up

15. Remove from the oven and place the cake pan onto a cooling metal rack for around 10 minutes.
16. Carefully take the cake out of the pan and place it onto the wire rack to cool thoroughly.
17. Cut the cake into serving portions and enjoy.

Tiramisu

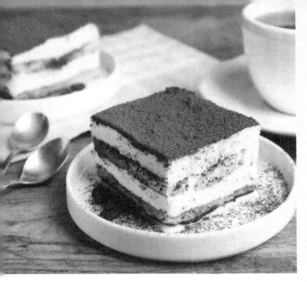

Prep period: 15 mins.
Cook period: 0 mins.
Serves: 9

Per Serving: Calories 199, Fat 6.3g
Carbs 26.1g, Protein 7.8g

INGREDIENTS REQUIRED:

- Heavy cream – ½ C. (120 g)
- Vanilla yogurt – 2 C. (500 g)
- Whole milk – 1 C. (240 ml)
- Brewed espresso – ½ C. (120 ml), cooled
- Crisp ladyfinger cookies – 24
- Baking cocoa – for dusting

PROCEDURE:

1. Put the cream into a small-siz basin and whisk to form stiff peaks.
2. Lightly blend in yogurt.
3. Put ½ C. of the cream mixtur the bottom of an 8-inch squar dish.
4. Put the milk and espresso int a shallow dish and blend to incorporate.
5. Dip 12 ladyfinger cookies int the espresso mixture, allowin the excess to drip off.
6. Place the dipped ladyfinger cookies over the cream mixtu
7. Top with half of the remnant cream mixture and dust with cocoa powder.
8. Repeat the layers.
9. Cover the baking pan and pu it into your fridge for at least hours before enjoying it.

Lime Cheesecake

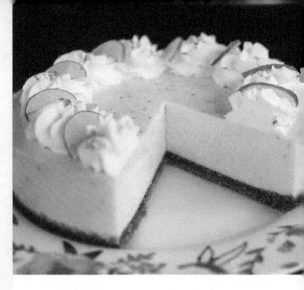

Prep period: 15 mins.

Cook period: 1 hr. 23 mins.

Serves: 12

er Serving: Calories 481, Fat 34.3g, Carbs 37.1g, Protein 8g

PROCEDURE:

For preheating: set your oven at 375 °F (190 °C).

For the crust, put the graham cracker crumbs and cinnamon into a basin and blend them thoroughly. Put in butter and blend to form a crumbly mixture.

Place the crumb mixture into a 10-inch springform pan and press into an even layer in the bottom and halfway up the sides of the pan.

Bake for around 7-8 minutes.

Again, set your oven at 375 °F (190 °C).

In the meantime, put the cream cheese into a basin and whisk to form a smooth texture.

Put in sugar and whisk to form a smooth mixture.

Put in sour cream, eggs, flour, and vanilla extract and whisk to form a smooth mixture.

Put in lime juice and blend to incorporate.

Place the filling mixture over the crust.

Bake for around 15 minutes.

Now, set your oven to 250 °F.

Bake for around 50 minutes.

Take the springform pan out of the oven and place it onto a cooling metal rack to cool for around 45-60 minutes.

Put it into your fridge for at least 6 hours before enjoying it.

INGREDIENTS REQUIRED:

For the Crust:
- Graham cracker crumbs – 2 C. (170 g), crushed
- Unsalted butter – ½ C. (110 g) liquefied
- White sugar – ¼ C. (50 g)

For the Filling:
- Cream cheese – 3 (8-oz.) (225-g) packages, softened
- White sugar – 1 C. (200 g)
- Sour cream – 1 C. (240 g)
- All-purpose flour – ¼ C. (35 g)
- Vanilla extract – 2 tsp. (10 ml)
- Eggs – 4
- Lime juice – ¾ C. (180 ml) freshly squeezed

NOTES

CONCLUSION

The Mediterranean diet is more than just a way of eating—it's a lifestyle rooted in centuries of tradition. Known for its rich flavors and health benefits, it emphasizes fresh vegetables, whole grains, lean proteins, and healthy fats. It has long been associated with improved well-being, reduced risk of heart disease, and a healthier, more balanced way of life.

This cookbook is your guide to bringing the essence of the Mediterranean diet into your own home. From satisfying breakfasts to indulgent desserts, each recipe is thoughtfully crafted to be both delicious and nourishing. Whether you're aiming for healthier meals or simply looking to expand your culinary skills, this book offers something for every taste. Now is the perfect time to discover how these simple, wholesome recipes can transform your meals and your health.

Made in the USA
Las Vegas, NV
04 January 2025

15847498R00079